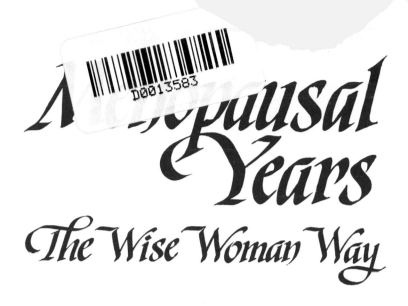

# New Menopausal Years
## The Wise Woman Way

### Susun S. Weed

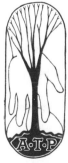

## Ash Tree Publishing
Woodstock, New York

All information in this *Wise Woman Ways* book is based on the experiences and research of the author and other professional healers. This information is shared with the understanding that you accept complete responsibility for your own health and well-being. You have a unique body. The action of every remedy is unique. Health care is full of variables. The result of any treatment suggested herein cannot always be anticipated and never guaranteed. The author and publisher are not responsible for any adverse effects or consequences resulting from the use of any remedies, procedures, or preparations included in this *Wise Woman Ways* book. Consult your inner guidance, knowledgeable friends, and trained healers in addition to the words written here.

Copyright © 1992 by Susun S. Weed.

Ash Tree Publishing, PO Box 64, Woodstock, NY 12498.
Phone/FAX: 914-246-8081

Typesetting by Kent Babcock.

Illustrations on pages 50, 122, 123, 180 © 1992 by Martha McGehee.

Cover calligraphy and illustrations on pages *xix*, 36, 42, 66, 87, 108, 118, 165, 172 © 1992 by Alan McKnight.

All other illustrations, including borders © by Susun Weed.

Please write for permission before reproducing any graphics in this book.

Printed and bound in the United States of America.

Library of Congress Catalog Card Number: 92-70069

ISBN 9614620-4-3

May the seven directions empower this medicine work.
May it be pleasing to my grandmothers, the ancient ones.
And may it be of benefit to all beings.

*So mote it be.*

# Acknowledgments

Many hearts and minds joined with mine to bring you this book. Here's where they step forward and take a bow.

The trees who gave themselves to make the paper . . . I thank you.

Alan McKnight who did (and did, and did) the cover illustration . . . I thank you.

Peggy Goddard who adroitly pasted up the boards . . . I thank you.

Chava Granett and Margriet Kreutzer and Mireille van Waaft who carefully did the index . . . I thank you.

Betsy Sandlin who edited magically in the midst of her Change . . . I thank you.

Cynthia Werthamer who edited so skillfully despite my stubbornness . . . I thank you.

Keyawis Kaplan who shares her angelic energy so magnificently with us all . . . I thank you.

Those who shared their stories of Change with me: my mom, Monica Shaft, and her cronies Hortense Bugbee and Kay Calvert; my aunts, Vicki Carlson, Yolanda Kowlowski, and Marianna Quigley; and the sisters of the sacred spiral, present and past . . . I thank you.

Those who read the work in progress and offered advice, encouragement, and criticism: Candace Cave who read it at sea, Holly (and David) Eagle who offered invaluable insights from their practice, Linda Dian Feldt and Penny King and Juliette de Baïracli Levy and Betsy Sandlin whose wise words shifted priorities and smoothed away rough edges, Pela Sander who lavished her expertise on this project, Marie Summerwood who kept me laughing, and Wonshé who — as always — helped me remember and believe . . . I thank you.

Those who helped me with research, massage, and their wholehearted excitement: Celu Amberston, Paul Bergner, Miriam Dyack, Lynn DeFilipo, Rosemary Gladstar, Jessica Godino, James Green, Belinda Hankins, Fern Hill, Brianna Kale, Liz Klipper, Gay Luce, Bruce MacFarland, Deborah Maia, Naryani, Christine Northrup, Melissa Oliphant, Judy Scher, Sylett Strickland, and Bob Walberg . . . I thank you.

And most especially, Michael Dattorre and Justine Swede, my mate and my daughter, who continually support my life and my work with their hearts, their minds, and their hands . . . I thank you.

# Introduction
### Juliette de Baïracli Levy

I am very pleased to write this introduction to Susun's excellent and much-needed book for the menopausal years. I hope it will go a long way toward changing those things that threaten the health and happiness of women today. It seems to me that the beauty and power of female life is too frequently cut away with hysterectomies and mastectomies nowadays. And too many women are encouraged to become dependent on costly and harmful chemical medications derived from cruel experiments on animals.

All the herbs and remedies I would like to see for the benefit and protection of women during their menopausal years are here, all in the right place and proportions. For example, I love lavender, one of the greatest of helps to us females from childhood to old age. And there it is, on page 90, perfectly described and used. And the Artemisias, those lovely plants named after the goddess Artemis, protector of all women, especially those birthing, are here as well.

This book shows very well Susun's great knowledge of herbs; she is clearly an herbalist deeply informed by her quarter century of intimate dialogues with people, plants, and animals. She has been using my herbals, "Common Herbs for Natural Health" and "Herbal for Farm and Stable" for decades and helping pass on the knowledge I collected from my encounters with "man and beast." I consider her one of the mothers of herbal medicine in the United States.

It is further flattery, but true! Susun Weed is a gifted writer. Her Crone passages, in which the old woman is giving advice and encouragement, often possess poetical beauty.

Susun is very well read on matters pertaining to the life and health of women. Her reference and resource lists, found throughout Wise Woman Ways for the Menopausal Years, are comprehensive and important.

This book should be in the hands of every woman, of every race, no matter what age, worldwide. I wish it the great success that it surely deserves.

# Table of Contents

# What Are the Menopausal Years?

Human females are unique from all other females on two counts (at least): we menstruate; and we cease to be reproductively available after we've lived only half of our life span. (Estrus bleeding in dogs is not menstruation.) The ancient women's mysteries tell us of the powers and initiations of these unique events: menstruation and menopause. This book focuses on the latter — the years of transformation from potential mother to wise, whole crone — the menopausal years.

Meno (*menstruation*) pause (*stops*) is, technically, the last menstrual flow of a woman's life. The years just before and just after the menopause itself are referred to as the *climacteric*. For most women the climacteric spans from early/mid 40s to late 50s/early 60s, including the premenopausal years, the menopausal climax years, and the post-menopausal years. To most of us, this entire period constitutes the menopausal years, popularly known as the **Change** of Life.

This **Change** is a metamorphosis (complete change at a cellular level). This metamorphosis follows, and may even be the matrix for, the three classic stages of initiation: isolation, death, and rebirth/reintegration. Each woman's **Change** includes these three stages, as well as three phases (before menopause, during menopause, and after menopause).

Each stage and phase of our metamorphic, menopausal **Change** is different; each has special needs and offers special challenges.

## Wise Woman Ways
## Premenopausal Years

The actual age at which menopausal **Change** begins varies considerably from woman to woman; the norm is 45, with a normal range of 35 to 55. During these premenopausal years, menstrual periods may become noticeably different (closer together, further apart, scantier, more profuse). Night sweats or hot flashes come, if at all, only occasionally and are usually blamed on too many blankets or a rich meal.

☞ **Nourish and tonify your entire hormonal system.** Menopausal changes occur not only in the ovaries, but also in the adrenal, thyroid, pancreas, pineal, and pituitary glands. Herbal allies are remarkably safe and effective glandular nourishers.

☞ **Increase the number and amount of calcium-rich foods you consume.** No single effort will repay you more richly. High levels of calcium in the diet protect you from osteoporosis, heart disease, and emotional swings. Green leafy vegetables (herbs and weeds) are exceptional sources of calcium.

☞ **Maintain regular menses.** Non-ovulatory menstrual cycles, common during the premenopausal years, lack a progesterone surge. Lack of progesterone contributes enormously to loss of bone mass and vaginal atrophy. Herbal allies can support progesterone production.

☞ **Find some regular physical activity to fall in love with.** Even gentle exercise, done regularly, helps maintain peak bone mass, strengthens the cardiovascular system, and insures deep sleep.

☞ **Gain up to a pound a year for ten years.** Thin women have more hot flashes and an altogether more difficult menopause than heavier women. Fat cells produce estrone, a kind of estrogen. (If you won't let yourself gain ten pounds, at least stop trying to lose weight. Dieting decreases bone mass and weakens the heart.)

☞ **Plan your Crone's Time Away.** The initial step of your initiation is isolation. As menopausal **Change** picks up speed at the end of the premenopausal years, many women find themselves desperate to be alone. Planning now can help make it a reality when you need it. Like an extended visit to the moonlodge (a sacred space where menstruating women can be away from daily life), Crone's Time Away is time when the menopausal woman is freed from all social responsibility and encouraged to tend solely to herself. An extended vacation, sabbatical or Crone's Year Away is ideal, but you can stay home and still take Crone's Time Away.

## Wise Woman Ways
## Menopausal Climax Years

The menopausal climax years include the year or two before and a year or more after your very last menstruation. The average age of a woman in the midst of her **Change** is 51.

But women come to their menopausal climax in their 20s, 30s, and 40s, as well. Some achieve menopause by surgical means, some by way of chemotherapy or radiation, and some just naturally arrive early. (Menopausal climax before the age of 40 is considered "premature.")

During this 2-5 year climax period, the bones refuse to take in calcium and bone scans will show growing osteoporosis; flashes, flushes, and night sweats may be frequent; palpitations, emotional sensitivity, and sleeplessness are common. Depending on the individual woman and her circumstances, other physical and emotional changes may come with the **Change**, or she may experience next to nothing.

☞ **Take time for solitude.** Although many women feel enormous satisfaction in tending and nurturing others, as our reproductive years come to a close, it is appropriate to turn away from care-taking. Hot flashes, sleeplessness, moodiness, and the like are easier to recognize as allies of wholeness when you are free to follow your own needs without concern for others. Take one day to be totally by yourself, or a Crone's Year Away, or anything in between.

☞ **Experiment with eggs, meat, and butter in your diet.** Some women find these foods, especially if from organic sources, *decrease* menopausal symptoms. Some practitioners insist they increase menopausal distress, especially when from commercial sources.

☞ **Relax and enjoy your hot flashes.** Ride them like waves, feel them in your spine, ski the edge of your flushes, honor the volcanic heat of your core. Like labor pains, hot flashes are the outward sign of metamorphosis. Like labor pains, they are worse when resisted. Herbal allies help those with unrelenting flashes relax and enjoy, too.

☞ **Spend time with a journal.** Buy a blank book and write in it, draw in it, paste articles in it. Visions and dreams are particularly vivid and intense in the menopausal climax years; keep your journal handy so you can record them. Your emotional energies are readily available during the menopausal climax years; draw them in your book. Memories abound during these years; cherish them in your journal. Write your autobiography.

☞ **Plan your Crone's Crowning.** As months pass and the moon waxes and wanes without drawing forth your menses, you pass through the second stage of initiation, death. Your identity as Mother dies. Let yourself break all the rules. Be someone totally different than you thought you could be.

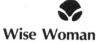

## Wise Woman Ways
## Post-Menopausal Years

The post-menopausal years symbolically begin on the fourteenth new moon after your final menstruation. (And continue, of course, for the rest of your life.) Hot flashes, aching joints, heart disease, incontinence, vaginal atrophy, and broken hips may diminish the quality and quantity of these years. Use of Wise Woman ways in the post-menopausal years can halt and reverse osteoporosis (the bones accept calcium once again), keep estrogen- and progesterone-sensitive tissues in the vagina and bladder from weakening and drying out, and maintain a healthy, vigorous heart and circulatory system.

☞ **Eat vegetables, fruits, and grains instead of meat.** Eating meat and meat fat weakens your bones as well as your heart, promotes cancer, and may contribute to post-menopausal hot flashes.

☞ **Move, dance, walk, stretch, go, inquire, keep active.** The essence of vitality is change. Now that you've been through the **Change**, don't stop, keep changing. Break the rules and the taboos. Become an expert on pelvic floor exercises. Take up belly dancing. Pump iron. Wear purple.

☞ **Write a legal will.** And revise it every ten years. Face your own death. Plan for your own death. This completes the second stage of your initiation.

☞ **Nourish yourself with every bite.** Aging increases our needs for many nutrients while reducing our digestive ability. Make every bite count toward optimum vitality and step up digestive efficiency by using dandelion root tincture before meals. Discover new ways to serve yourself calcium-rich foods at every meal. Use herbal vinegars regularly. Gradually replace bone-depleting white flour products (bread, pasta, pretzels) with fiber-rich whole grains and whole grain products. Drink vitamin- and mineral-rich herbal infusions instead of mineral-depleting coffee, tea, and soft drinks. Try yogurt and fresh fruit instead of ice cream for stronger bones and fewer vaginal infections.

☞ **Plan your Crone's Ceremony of Commitment to Her Community.** Anytime after your second Saturn return (age 57-61), you are ready for the third stage of your menopausal initiation: rebirth. You are She-Who-Holds-the-Wise-Blood-Inside. You are newly crowned, newly born, baby Crone. After isolation, after death, you rejoin the community. In your isolation, you revisioned yourself. By giving death to yourself as Mother, you claimed all of yourself. It is time to share that vision, to name yourself publicly, Crone, woman of wholeness.

*"I am the Crone. I feel my way along paths following the energy and warmth that others have placed here. Trusting the dark, I am guided not by light, but by the flowing movements I sense. I am like the water that follows, without sight or foreknowledge, the ancient river's channel."*

My Native American teachers tell me that we are in the midst of earth changes that will culminate around the year 2013. They say the earth changes will bring heat, and floods, and upheaval on an enormous scale. I am struck by the fact that more than 50 million women will have achieved menopause by 2013. Since we, as women, are one with the Earth, is our massive, collective **Change** her **Change** as well? Can we moderate her hot flashes? Give her ease from flooding? Soothe her emotional uproar? Emerge transformed together after our changes? How will we do it? With drugs, against the problems? With nature, blessed by all we are given? Will it matter to the Earth, Gaia, what choices I make in my menopause? What stories I tell myself? What I tell other women?

## Hormonal Changes Before, During, & After Menopause

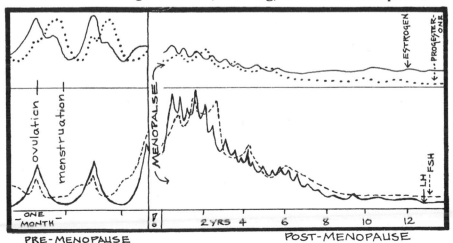

# The Six Steps of Healing

(Parentheses suggest a few of the modalities of each step.)

*Step 0: Do nothing* (sleep, meditate, unplug the clock or the telephone). A vital, invisible step.

*Step 1: Collect information* (low-tech diagnosis, reference books, support groups, divination).

*Step 2: Engage the energy* (prayer, homeopathic remedies, crying, visualizations, ritual, aromatherapy, color, laughter).

*Step 3: Nourish and tonify* (herbal infusions/vinegars, love, some herbal tinctures, life-style changes, physical activities, moxibustion).

*Step 4: Stimulate/Sedate* (hot/cold water, many herbal tinctures, acupuncture, most massage, alcohol). Risk of developing dependence on step 4 remedies is influenced by frequency (how often), dosage (how much), and duration (how long).

*Step 5a: Use supplements* (synthesized/concentrated vitamins or minerals, special foods like royal jelly or spirulina). Supplements are *not* step 3. There's always the risk with synthesized/concentrated substances that they'll do more harm than good, e.g., the men who took fish liver oil in capsules and had a greater mortality from heart disease (the oil was rancid).

*Step 5b: Use drugs* (synthesized alkaloids, oral and injectable hormones, high dilution homeopathics). Overdose may cause grave injury or death.

*Step 6: Break and enter* (fear-inspiring language, surgery, colonics, Rolfing, psychoactive drugs, invasive "diagnostic" tests such as mammograms and biopsies). Side effects are inevitable and may include permanent injury or death.

# Using This Book

• Start by looking through the whole book quickly. Life is not neatly divided into chapters. Each woman will achieve her menopause in her own unique and individual way. My broad divisions of premenopausal, menopausal, and post-menopausal may not fit your experiences. *Any of the remedies may be used at any time in one's life.*

• Pay particular attention to Appendix 2. The results and safety of any remedy are dependent on your ability to prepare it appropriately and use it appropriately. Note that I use **herbal vinegars** and **herbal infusions**, which are quite different from culinary vinegars and herbal teas.

• Look through the remedies for your problem. I've arranged the remedies from safest to most dangerous, using as my pattern the Six Steps of Healing in the Wise Woman way. Step 0 is the safest; step 6, the most dangerous.

★ If you want something that works well, and the sooner the better, look for the stars marking my favorite remedies. Most of them are remedies that many women have used with favorable results.

• Use steps 0, 1, 2, and 3 as preventive medicine. Prevention is an important, though often invisible, way of healing/wholing in the Wise Woman tradition. You're never too old to need deep relaxation, information, energetic engagement, nourishment (that includes love), and exercise.

• If you want to remedy your problem with the least possible side effects and danger, start at step 1. (Whether or not I mention it as a specific remedy, step 0 is always appropriate.) After reading step 1, pick one remedy from step 2 and set a time limit for working with it. If your problem is unresolved within that time, decide if the time limit needs expanding or if you are ready to go to step 3. Continue in this manner, moving to steps 4, 5, or 6 as needed, until your problem is solved. Each step up increases the possibility of side effects and their severity, so I strongly urge you to try at least one of the step 2 techniques, even if they seem strange to you, before going on to the remedies of steps 3 and beyond. (Note also that time spent at step 2 will help you choose appropriate remedies at step 3, and so on.) When your problem is resolved, don't stop. Go back through the steps, in reverse, before resting at step 0.

• You can continue to take remedies from a previous step after moving on, but be cautious about the use of step 4 remedies in combination with step 5 remedies. Motherwort tincture and vitamin E (5a) may be fine together, while valerian and an antidepressant (5b) may not. (See next section: "Using Herbs Safely.")

• If you deem it necessary to heal through step 5 and/or 6 (and real healing can and does take place with the aid of drugs and surgery) and have not yet tried any techniques from steps 2 and 3, do so immediately. Engaging the energy, nourishing and tonifying will aid and abet the healing powers of the more dangerous healing ways and help prevent or moderate their side effects.

• Note that Appendix 2 lists food/herb sources of all vitamins and minerals (step 5a) needed during the menopausal years. If you are currently taking supplements, you may want to taper off and use more optimum sources of nourishment such as weeds and herbal infusions.

• Use the index to help you find more information on an herb you are using. Wise Woman teaching flows in spiraling cycles, so this book is not a formal garden with a *Materia Medica*, but rather a wildflower garden with different information on one plant appearing here and there throughout the book.

• Note that I have included German, French, and Chinese names for many herbal allies.

• Trust your own sense of what's right for *you*. Use this book in conjunction with your own inner Wise Woman. Seek second and third opinions. Respect the uniqueness of your body, your intuitions, and your feelings.

• May it be in beauty; may it be in a sacred way.

# Using Herbs Safely

Plants feed us, clothe us, house us, heal us, and kill us. There's no way around it, when you use herbs you need to be alert and aware. Here are some ways to be sure you're using herbs safely.

• Identify all plants you intend to use by botanical name (e.g. *Leonurus cardiaca*). Only buy herbs that are labeled with the botanical name. The botanical name is specific to only one plant, while common names overlap and vary. "Sage" refers to at least five plants in at least two different families, but *Salvia officinalis* only means garden sage.

• Use only one herb at a time. Learn all you can about that one herb. Read books; experiment on yourself, others, pets; listen to your elders' stories. If you discover that your herbal ally likes to work with partners, pair her up with other herbs one at a time.

• Seek out the worth of the weeds on your doorstep. Learn about, eat, or use as a remedy, one wild food/medicine that grows in your yard or nearby lot this year. When you make your own medicines and healing foods you eliminate one of the possible dangers of crude herb use: mistaken identity (or right label, wrong herb). Not that you can't make mistakes, but you're more likely to catch your own mistake than someone else's. When you make your own medicines and healing foods, they are fresh, full of energy, and in tune with you and your environment. You'll also feel better as you become more aware of the vitality and abundance of nature expressing herself everywhere.

• Begin with gentle nourishing and tonifying herbal infusions and vinegars. Watch carefully for side effects during the first 24 hours the first time you use any new plant. But don't worry if it takes your system a couple of tries to figure out how to digest a new food/herb. Use herbal tinctures after you have some grounding in the use of herbs as foods and infusions. Start with the smaller recommended dose and build up slowly if you need.

• Build up a foundation of trust in the healing effectiveness of plants by using remedies for minor problems before tackling serious concerns.

• Gather or join a support group of people interested in self-care and home remedies and consult them when you feel uncertain.

• Respect the power of plants; those strong enough to act as stimulants, sedatives, and near-drugs (such as opium) affect the body and spirit in powerful ways and may be useful only in minute doses.

• Respect the unique individuality of every plant, every person, every situation.

• Remember that you become whole and healed in your own unique way, as you will. Plants can help in this process. People can help in this process. (Animals, too.) But each individual body/spirit does the healing/wholing itself. Don't expect plants to be cure-alls.

• Respect the differences between herbs used in step 3 — nourishing and tonifying herbs — and those used in steps 4 and 5 — stimulating, sedating, and toxic herbs.

**Nourishing herbs** are the safest of all herbs; side effects are quite rare. Nourishing herbs may generally be taken in any quantity for any period of time. They are foods, just as leafy greens, garlic, and carrots are. They provide high-level nutrients, including vitamins, minerals, trace minerals, starches, simple and complex sugars, bioflavonoids, carotenes, and essential fatty acids (EFAs). The nourishing herbs in *Wise Woman Ways for the Menopausal Years* are: alfalfa, borage, calendula, chamomile, chickweed, cornsilk, comfrey, elder blossoms or berries, fennel, fenugreek, lemon balm, mallows, nettles, oatstraw, plantain, raspberry, red clover, seaweeds, sweet briar (rose hips), St. Joan's wort (*Hypericum*), slippery elm, and violet.

**Tonifying herbs** act slowly in the body and have a cumulative, rather than immediate, effect. They are most beneficial when they are used in small quantities for extended periods of time. Side effects are slightly more common with tonics. (Note that many herbalists equate stimulating herbs with the tonics, leading to misuse and unwanted side effects.) The more bitter the tonic tastes, the less you need to take of it. Bland tonics may be used like nourishing herbs, in quantity. Nearly half of the herbs in *Wise Woman Ways for the Menopausal Years* are tonics, including: birch, black cohosh, blackstrap molasses, chaste tree, dandelion, Dong Quai/Dang Gui, echinacea, false unicorn, ginseng, hawthorn, horsetail, lady's mantle, motherwort, peony, sarsaparilla, spikenard, wild yam, and yellow dock.

**Sedating/Stimulating herbs** cause a wide variety of usually rapid reactions, some of which may be unwanted. Long-term use can lead to dependency, so sedating/stimulating herbs are best used in moderate doses for fairly short periods of time. Side effects are frequent; there may be loss of tone or a rebound/manic effect when the herb is no longer taken. Some parts of the person may be stressed in order to help other parts. The sedating/stimulating herbs in *Wise Woman Ways for the Menopausal Years* are: catnip, cinnamon, ginger, hops, licorice, myrrh, passion flower, poplar, primrose, sage, skullcap, uva ursi, valerian, vervain, willow, and wintergreen.

**Toxic herbs** are potential poisons and potent medicines. They activate intense effort on the part of the body and spirit. Toxic herbs are taken in tiny amounts for very short periods of time. Unexpected side effects are common when toxic herbs are used without regard for their power. Increase your herbal knowledge and sense of security when contemplating use of a toxic herb by consulting other herbal references and several experienced herbalists. It is especially important to check on the possible side effects of toxic herbs if you are allergic to any foods or medicines. The toxic herbs in *Wise Woman Ways for the Menopausal Years* are: cayenne, cotton root, goldenseal, liferoot, poke root, rue, sweet clover (*Melilot*), and wormseed.

**Green blessings.**

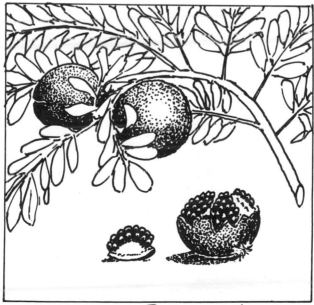

Pomegranate — *Punica granatum*

# Foreword
## Wonshé (Sher Willis)

I first read this book at the time of my own quickening as Crone. I was experiencing biological changes, shifts in my rhythm that I had never known, yet somehow remembered. These changes were deep, primal; they called me to respond to everything from a visceral place. I was a volcano ready to erupt, a bird destroying her own nest, an island about to form. Friends and practitioners insisted I was too young (not yet 40) to be menopausal. I felt like a woman, pregnant for the first time, who has never seen another pregnant woman.

Then *Wise Woman Ways for the Menopausal Years* came to my hands. Susun's words affirmed my Change, brought my opposites together, showed me how to use all my healing options wisely, and offered me an unsurpassed opportunity to recreate my wholeness.

As a midwife, and keeper of the blood mysteries, I see a profound parallel between the experiences of menopause and those of child-bearing. As Crone, or as Mother, we generate power from the arche-typal and elemental source of all life: female sexual energy.

With the help of *Wise Woman Ways for the Menopausal Years*, we can use this energy to resanctify ourselves, to re-wild ourselves, and to break free from the unnatural definitions of menopause that would domesticate and disempower us.

As an herbal resource alone, it is of extensive value to every reader. And it is more than just a book about menopause. It speaks to our entire planet — literally, symbolically, scientifically, poetically, authen-tically — from the heart of a wise woman. It is perhaps the single most important book for women — and men — to read as we move toward the turn of the century and the time of the "earth changes." Woven throughout the text is the ancient truth of the new millenium of our planet: the potent image of woman reflecting the spirit and truth of Earth as Earth reflects the truth and spirit of woman.

Thank you sister. Thank you Susun. Now I understand what meno-pause is: a time to generate female sexual energy beyond fertility, a season to Change with Earth, and an initiation.

# Preface

February cold rainbows glint in mooncaught snow. My birthday. This is the face of an aging woman who looks at me, clear-eyed, from my mirror. This is a face which has known some weathers: smiles line the mouth and eyes, worries are gathered between the brows, and forty-six winters glitter silver lights (like the rainbows in the snow under the full moon) from my crown. Forty-six is surely not yet old. But just as surely getting old. Old woman. Getting to be an old woman.

Now my monthly bleeding is precious. Dear. Soon I will go without it. The anxious wait for blood to signal that I am *not* pregnant turns on its head and becomes an anxious wait for blood to show that I *am* still fertile. This companion of more than thirty years is preparing to leave; I feel her restless stirrings, the way her attention wanders, how irregular she's become. I know my life will be different when she's gone.

Different? How? Without my monthly bloody show will I be a woman? Is this not what made me a woman when I thought I was but a girl? All I know of myself as woman is the ripening of the egg, the building of the nest, the giving unto/into life.

*"Great granddaughter, it is time to prepare for your journey. I am Grandmother Growth. I, my plant friends, and my stories have come to guide you on your menopausal journey, your metamorphosis to Crone, woman of wholeness."*

Crone? Old woman! Change? The **Change**! Menopause! When my ovaries abandon me to the ravages of old age: brittle bones! uncertain heart! withered sexuality! wrinkles! grey hair! No!

Why do I wake at night sweating? Bad dreams? Too many covers? Hot flash? Hot flash! But I'm too young. I'm bleeding. It can't be. I'm not ready. Hot flash? How can I keep up my work? Maintain my responsibilities? Hot flash! Oh no.

*"I bring you the ancient women's mystery stories. Take the time to listen to me. Slow down. Take time off so you can hear the old, old memories beginning to chant in your bones, drum in your heart, pulse in your veins, transform your energy."*

*The Crone reaches out her hand. The air crackles with heat and power, a sudden sweat starts up along your sides, between your thighs, around your neck, along your spine. The sensation is intense.*

*"Open your hands; release your expectations. Take my hand. Let me awaken memories of wise old women, crazy old women, peaceful, joyous, strong, invisible old women, whose trail you can find and walk, whose songs you can hear and sing. Journey with me into Change, sing with me the forgotten melodies, come with me along this old, old trail. Come, baby Crone, come."*

Modern western doctors and the media tell me I'm on my way over the hill; that I should prepare for the inevitable downhill slide. "Your ovaries are calling it quits," they tell me. "Soon you'll be a useless old woman. Your bones will break, your heart will fail, and all because you're lacking estrogen. Of course, we can supply you with it . . . for a price. And any price is worth paying for your share of estrogen. It may cost you your breasts and your uterus, but at least you'll still be a woman."

Grandmother, what is happening? Everything seems so strange. I thought I was comfortable with myself in many forms, but I don't know who I am any more. What is overcoming me? What am I becoming?

*"Sweet child, the wise woman achieves menopause, it does not overcome her. Through the gate of menopause the wise woman steps into her final glory, her crowning as Crone. Daughter, sister, listen well: the time and place in which you live seeks to deny you your last crown. Few leaders and healers of your day honor the Crone. Instead, they try to beguile you with the flowery wreath of the Maiden or the Mother's lush harvest headdress, telling you that growth into your deep maturity, into your Cronehood, is not worthwhile, not desirable; you must stay young. They hope to scare you away from this powerful Change, to convince you it's a deficiency state, of all things. Come with me and learn the true nature of your metamorphosis to Crone, woman of wholeness."*

Grandmother Growth, if I go with you, if I sing with you, if I ally with your plant friends, will it be an easy journey?

*"Not even I can promise you that, granddaughter. The journey of each woman into and through menopause is unique. If you encounter harsh weather or unexpected setbacks . . . well, that is the truth of the journey."*

Ovary, ovary, talk to me. What are you doing? Are you tired? Out of juice? energy? eggs? Ovary, ovary, both of you, say something for yourselves. Are we still in this together?

"Woman, it is well that you sit in silence and hark to our words. Here in your ovaries there are memories. In the womb of your mother we gathered these memories, memories passed down from mother egg to daughter egg for hundred of thousands of years. It is true that our stock of eggs grows low. This is as it should be, for our store of memories is full.

"Just as we have released ripened eggs each month, flooding your system with hormones so you could conceive and gestate, now we begin to release memories and the hormones needed to gestate memories. Take the time to ripen and swell these memories and you can give birth to the past (which, incidentally, changes the future).

"With our help, you have held out the hand of **giving life** for many years. Let it rest now. Come to know the hand of **giving death**. Grasp the hand of Grandmother Growth, grasp the fact of your own death. And thus anchored in reality, give death to yourself as Maiden, give death to yourself as Mother, and birth yourself as Crone, woman of wholeness, who enfolds and holds within herself Maiden, Mother, and Crone, life and death."

Grandmother Growth suddenly appears, and drops a quartz crystal into my upturned palm.

*"Now, great granddaughter. Take my hand. Yes, release the crystal, let it roll into the stream. Let go of yourself as Maiden. Take my hand."*

Her gaze holds my eyes, which are suddenly wet with tears. Something small and cool slides into my palm. *"Take my hand."* I glance quickly down to see light shimmering in my hand.

*"Let go of the moonstone, too. Nest it into the earth at the base of this tree. Let go of yourself as Mother. Take the hand of Grandmother Growth and open your eyes, wide. Look here. What do you see?"*

Yes, this is the face of an aging woman who looks at me, clear-eyed, from my mirror. A woman walking toward herself as Crone. A woman humming the long-forgotten songs of menopause. An aging woman with many questions.

February cold rainbows glint in mooncaught snow. My birthday. For years I have dreamt about and researched menopause.

*"It is time to share."*

It is time to share what I have uncovered, discovered, recovered. I offer, through these words, the guidance of my own heart and inner wisdom as well as the results of my studies.

*"Take my hand."*

Yes, take my hand, and walk a ways with me, and share my excitement at the *Menopausal Years*.

SSW
Laughing Rock Farm
8 February 1992

# MENOPAUSAL GODDESS

Described as a "snake or bird woman, Goddess of inspiration and creative energy, 4500BC," this figure – and the many others like it - may portray a menopausal woman having a hot flash.

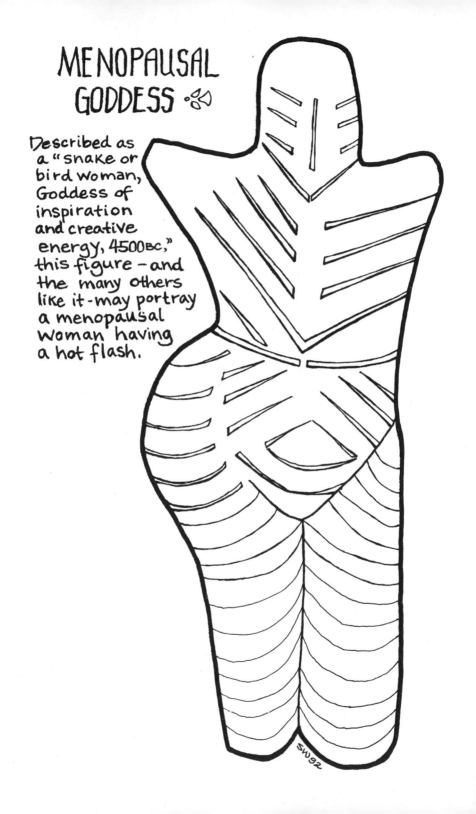

SW92

# Is This Menopause?
## Preparing for the Journey

*"Is today not the best day to begin?" asks Grandmother Growth. "If you are old enough to ask 'Is this menopause?,' you are old enough to plan your journey to the old woman you are growing into. Let us gather what we need. It is time to begin your journey into Change."*

"Is this menopause?" is a self-answering question. As soon as you ask, consider the process begun. Something is changing or you wouldn't be asking. Irregular periods? An occasional hot flash? If you are over forty, you are definitely beginning your menopausal years. (Menopausal changes begin for some women even earlier.)

"Is this menopause?" It is the rare woman who menstruates every 28 days until one month she simply doesn't any more. For most of us, menopause is a process that takes many years, not a specific, knowable end-point.

"Is this menopause?" In linear time, in the minds of many MDs and gynecologists, menopause is a single event, a definite end: the last menses. But to the wise woman, to the woman experiencing menopause, menopause is a spiraling process over time.

"Is this menopause?" you surmise as you skip a cycle, then bleed normally for a year.

"Is this menopause?" you ponder, struggling to understand your new sexual preferences and appetites.

"Is this menopause?" you desperately hope as the blood pulses out of you in torrents.

"Is this menopause?" Since you asked: Yes, it is. And there are preparations you can make *now* that will help ease your journey of **Change**, of transformation, of initiation as a fully mature woman.

"Is this menopause?" you wonder, taking off your sweater when everyone else seems chilled.

"Is this menopause?" you guess as you start to bleed 13 days after your last menses.

Yes, this is menopause. Your menopausal years have begun. Ally with hormone-balancing herbs, now. They'll moderate menopausal flooding and stabilize the ending of your menstrual cycles. They'll nourish and tonify the glands in transition at menopause, so you can encounter your flashes (of heat! of insight!) with more serenity.

"Is this menopause?" you think as you awaken, feeling sweaty, and toss off the covers.

"Is this menopause?" you wonder as you contemplate your first grey hairs . . . your first serious wrinkles . . . the softening texture of your skin . . . the way your breasts and belly give in more and more to the downward tug of gravity.

"Is this menopause?" you suspect as you find yourself sleeping less yet flowing with creative juices.

"Is this menopause?" you ask, noticing that you're digesting everything (food, people, events) differently.

"Is this menopause?" you whisper, feeling bone-tired, deathly tired, deeply exhausted.

This is menopause and you are not alone. This is menopause no matter what your doctor says. You are beginning your **Change** and you can change with ease and grace. Let herbs and other foods rich in essential fatty acids help you **Change**. They'll moderate cardiovascular disturbances (flashes, flushes, sweats), strengthen your liver, and help keep your energy level high and your heart healthy.

Let calcium-rich herbs and foods give you deeper sleep, more even emotions, and strong old bones. (The more bone mass built before the cessation of your menses, the more you'll have as a crone.)

The physical/menstrual/emotional/sexual changes that accompany menopause may be frightening. Let Grandmother Growth help. She knows the ways of women's mysteries. She lives the ways of the wise woman, healing and wholing person and planet. She offers stories about **Change**, new ways to understand the menopausal years, and new visions of old woman, She-Who-Holds-the-Wise-Blood-Inside.

*"Shall we begin?"*

# Menstrual Irregularities

*"Take heed, great granddaughter," murmurs Grandmother Growth. "You are growing and changing. Sometime soon you will achieve your menopause. Take time now to listen to your inner wise woman. Lend your inner ear to the voice of your uterus, your ovaries. Lend your heart to their urgent messages.*

*"Your blood is moving in new ways, dear woman," sings Grandmother Growth. "Resistance will only make you tired. Allow the movements and Changes inside you to spill out. There is no separation between your life and your Change. Let go now of your routines, your habits, your need for control. Give yourself up entirely to this Change, this seeming chaos. I promise you, it will only be for a short while."*

You may very well feel the first tremors of your **Change** in increasing menstrual changes. Your menstrual cycles may become erratic. You may find yourself passing large clots when you bleed. You may spot. It is a rare woman who simply stops having her regular periods, never to bleed again (though it does happen).

Irregular intervals between menses is the norm as you enter the menopausal years. The remedies offered here don't imply that we ought to have regular menses during the menopausal years. The erratic movements of our cycles help us transform our self-image from fertile woman/Mother to wise grandmother/Crone.

Large blood loss at menstruation and mid-cycle spotting are also normal during menopause. In a non-ovulatory cycle, the blood-rich lining of the uterus never gets a signal to stop growing. So it grows until the sheer bulk of it causes a menstrual flow/flood.

Since hysterectomy is frequently suggested to premenopausal women as a "life saving" measure, the remedies offered here for flooding (and fibroids, a frequent cause of flooding) are given in the hope of saving not only your life, but your uterus as well, that you may ever be a womb-one.

The quotes are from real women; may they help us remember that each woman's experience of menopause is uniquely her own.

# Erratic Intervals Between Flows

*"I never know when to expect my flow now. Sometimes it comes in two weeks, sometimes in six."*

### Step 1. Collect information . . .

Don't be surprised if your menstrual pattern changes noticeably sometime in your 40s (or late 30s). You may "skip" a cycle or two, find your menstrual bleeding scanty, or have heavier periods than you've ever had, sometimes two weeks apart. How can you tell what's normal and what's not?

Missing periods is fine. Missing periods for months and then getting them again is also fine. Very little blood and very much blood, even with big clots, is fine if it seems and feels like menstruation to you. (As in saying, when the blood shows: "Oh, that's why I was so irritable . . . constipated . . . weepy . . . [you name it] . . . yesterday.")

If the amount of blood is usual for you but the pattern is weird, that's menopause. If the cycle is usual for you, but the amount of blood isn't, that's menopause. If you seemingly skip a period and then have a real drencher several weeks later, that's menopause. If you spot or even bleed a bit at ovulation, that's menopause.

So, how can you distinguish the normal bleeding "abnormalities" of menopause from really abnormal bleeding needing attention and treatment?

Listen to your body. Pay attention to your dreams. Trust your own wisdom. Talk to other women. Keep records. I've charted my menstrual cycles for years on a Lunar Phases chart by Susan Baylies (Snake and Snake, Rt 3, Box 165, Durham, NC 27713 / $2) and recommend it highly. With thirteen months of moons on one sheet, your patterns, even during menopause, are easily seen. You may find a certain regularity to your irregularity.

Note: If what worries you about erratic menses in the premenopausal years is difficulty with birth control, see page 38.

• **It is always wise to seek the opinion of someone experienced in women's health care if you are bothered by erratic or profuse menses.**

### Step 2. Engage the energy . . .

• Sleep where the **full moon** can shine on your face if your menses are highly erratic. If that isn't possible, sleep in a totally dark room except for the three nights when the moon is full. On those nights, turn on a small light and sleep with it on all night.

• **Reduce stress.** Do a full-body relaxation before going to sleep.

• It takes a lot of energy to journey through menopause and you may feel "unreasonably" tired. **Take time for yourself when you bleed; plan your Crone's Time Away.**

### Step 3. Nourish and tonify . . .

• **Raspberry leaf** infusion, a cup or more a day, tonifies and nourishes the ovaries as well as the uterus, helping your **Change** flow smoothly.

★ **Dong Quai/Dang Gui Compound Tincture** (see page 194) warms, regulates, and gently heals the entire reproductive system; especially useful if your irregular cycles are accompanied by premenstrual distress.

• Tincture of **lifroot blossoms**, 5 drops taken daily, helps tonify the reproductive-hormone producers: ovaries, uterus, adrenals, liver, and pituitary.

• **Vitex** tincture is slow-acting, but highly recommended for the woman bothered by menopausal irregularities. Use a dropperful in a small glass of water or juice two or three times daily for six to eight weeks after every irregular period.

• Nothing tones the pelvic area and helps maintain regular menstruation — up until the very last period — like regular sexual stimulation and **release** (orgasm), alone or partnered. Pelvic-floor exercises (see page 134) are a close second, though.

★ One or more tablespoons/15 ml of fresh **wheat germ oil** added to the daily diet was the remedy used by savvy grandmothers fifty years ago to regulate menses, protect the heart and help keep the vagina lubricated. **Vitamin E oil** does the same.

### Step 4. Stimulate/Sedate . . .

★ **Reduce animal fats** in the diet. Animal fats are converted by the body into estrogens, thus confusing the delicate feedback mechanisms regulating your journey through menopause. (Animal fats may also contain supplemental hormones fed to the animals and passed along to you, further confusing your body wisdom.)

• **Cinnamon** (*Cinnamomum zeylanicum*) bark invigorates the blood, helps regulate the menstrual cycle, and checks flooding. Sip a cup/250 ml of infusion, use 5-10 drops of tincture once or twice a day, gnaw on a cinnamon stick, or simply sprinkle cinnamon powder on everything you eat. (*Everything?!*)

• **Acupuncture** is very effective in regulating erratic menses.

### Step 5b. Use drugs . . .

• Birth control pills are used to regulate menstrual intervals. While effective for women in their fertile years, this treatment is considered inappropriate for women past the age of forty, due to increasingly dangerous side effects from the synthetic hormones.

### Step 6. Break and enter . . .

*"After the last planned pregnancy, the uterus becomes a useless, bleeding, symptom-producing, potentially cancer-bearing organ and therefore should be removed."*                    –RC Wright, MD, gynecologist, 1988

• The modern scientific remedy for premenopausal problems such as erratic periods is simple and neat: remove the uterus! Without the uterus there is no worry about birth control or uterine cancer. (This makes it much safer for you to take estrogen replacement therapy.) A hysterectomy is major surgery. While loss of your uterus will not necessarily make you ill, retaining your uterus can contribute significantly to your self-image as a whole/healthy woman, as well as to your sexual, emotional, and physical health.

# Flooding

*"I would contrive to get two super tampons inside and I'd use two thick pads as well, but I couldn't make it through the night, and when I went to the bathroom I'd leave a trail of blood behind."*

### Step 1. Collect information . . .

Heavy bleeding (flooding) is common in menopausal and pre-menopausal women as a response to changing hormonal levels, most notably progesterone levels. A drop in progesterone signals the uterus to contract and expel the menses, so when progesterone levels stay high during the cycle, the endometrium continues to grow and reaches an unprecedented density and richness. It actually grows so dense that it crowds itself out of the uterus. When that finally happens, you have a "late" period that comes in floods, gushes, and clots.

Some healthy menopausal women report bleeding heavily for as long as 10-14 days. Midwives note that it isn't so much the actual amount of blood a woman loses as her physiological response to the blood loss. Weakness, dizziness, paleness, and mental confusion are danger signals.

Loss of blood always means loss of iron. And with intense blood loss comes iron deficiency, which aggravates blood loss. **Keep iron levels high.** (See page 8 and page 186.)

If the following remedies seem to have no effect, seek the advice of someone knowledgeable in the ways of women; consult with a gynecologist if you can. Flooding is also an indicator of uterine and ovarian distresses such as an irritation or infection from an IUD, fibroids, ovarian cysts, adenomatous hyperplasia, cervical/uterine/ endometrial polyps, or, rarely, cancer. Of these, only cancer is directly life-threatening. (Remedies for women with cysts, polyps, hyperplasia, and reproductive cancers are in my book *Wise Woman Ways for Women Who Love Their Breasts and Uterus and Don't Want to Lose Them*.)

**Seek knowledgeable advice and health care from an experienced person if your period lasts more than twice as long as it ever did, if you have pain or bleeding with intercourse, or if your flooding is accompanied by persistent low back/pelvic pain.**

### Step 2. Engage the energy . . .

★ One of the best homeopathic remedies for menopausal flooding is **Lachesis**. Use it when the blood is very dark, thick, and strong-smelling; when pain, if present, is more intense at the beginning of the flow; and when rage is the predominant emotion.

★ One of the most useful and deep-acting of the homeopathic remedies for heavy bleeding is **Sepia**. Try it when the periods come frequently, the bleeding is heavy, painful, and accompanied by backache or constipation, and depression.

• Other useful **homeopathic remedies** include:
  ☞ *Belladonna:* flooding with bright red blood and clots; you're swollen, ultra sensitive, and/or headachy before and during bleeding.
  ☞ *Ipecacuanha:* flooding is bright red and continuous; you may have cramps, feel weak, and/or vomit.
  ☞ *Secale:* flooding without clots, but with severe cramps.
  ☞ *Sabina:* severe cramping, weakness, clots accompany flooding.
  ☞ *China:* flooding with dark clots; exhaustion.
  ☞ *Crocus sativa:* flooding with clots but without pain.
  ☞ *Natrum mur.:* flooding brings tears, exhaustion, depression; periods irregular and prolonged; cramps, headache, constipation.
  ☞ *Sulfur:* for the woman who floods and has drenching sweats with hot flashes.

### Step 3. Nourish and tonify . . .

★ **Lady's mantle** (*Alchemilla vulgaris*), the alchemical weed, controlled menstrual hemorrhage in virtually all of more than 300 women in a recent study. When taken after flooding began, lady's mantle took 3-5 days to be effective. When taken for 1-2 weeks before menstruation, lady's mantle prevented flooding. Use 5-10 drops of the fresh plant tincture 3 times a day for up to two weeks out of the month.

★ The single most important element for the premenopausal woman who bleeds heavily is **iron**. Try to consume 2 mg or more of iron from herbs and foods each day you flood; 1-1.5 mg daily on days you aren't bleeding. Expect to feel more energetic and alive within two weeks. Flooding is usually noticeably diminished at the next menses.

The best source of usable iron is **dandelion leaves**. They contain 5+ mg in 1 ounce/30 grams. An alcohol or vinegar tincture of fresh **yellow dock root** is also excellent. A dose of 20 drops of alcohol tincture, or 3 teaspoons/15 ml vinegar, taken in tea or water, contributes more than 1 mg iron to the blood. (Other sources of iron on page 186.) Note that coffee, black tea, soy protein, egg yolks, bran, and calcium supplements over 250 mg impair iron absorption.

Take iron throughout the day, not in one big dose. Most bodies can only absorb a little iron at a time. To further enhance absorption, take it with some orange juice or milk. (Acids and proteins increase iron uptake.)

★ **Bioflavonoids** strengthen the capillaries and provide estrogenic factors; together these effects help decrease flooding. (See page 178.)

★ A lack of prostaglandins contributes to menopausal flooding. (And a surplus contributes to menopausal flashing!) Oils rich in gammalinoleic acid (GLA) are precursors to and balancers of prostaglandin production in the body. Raising GLA levels can help you decrease your flooding rapidly and substantially.

• **Flax seed** (*Linum usitatissimum*), also known as linseed, contains an oil unsurpassed in health benefits, but only if it is absolutely fresh and taken uncooked. Some women take 1-3 teaspoons/5-15 ml of flax seed oil first thing in the morning. Others grind the seeds and sprinkle them on their breakfast cereal or lunch salad. (Drink a glass of water or mug of herbal infusion at the same time, please.) Others soak flax seeds overnight in water and drink the whole thing (yes, eat the seeds) first thing in the morning. (Organic flax seed oil and powder available by mail from Omega Nutrition, 1720 La Bounty Rd, Ferndale, WA 98248.)

If you don't see results from daily use within a month, try using the oil pressed from the seeds of any one of these plants for a month: **borage** (*Borago officinalis*), **black currant** (*Ribes nigrum*), or **evening primrose** (*Oenothera biennis*). They are all high in GLA. Store and take the same way as flax seed oil.

★ **Vitex** berries, taken in tincture form, 25 drops several times daily for several months, will stabilize progesterone shifts and decrease flooding. Women whose normal menstrual flow is heavy may wish to begin using vitex immediately as its effect is slow to appear.

★ **Wild yam** root tincture, 20-30 drops taken daily for the two weeks preceding the expected onset of menses, can supply enough progesterone precursors to remedy flooding. (See step 5 below.)

• **Astringent uterine tonics** are often suggested for the woman bleeding profusely during her forties. My favorites are uva ursi, raspberry leaves, garden sage, and black haw bark. Infuse singly or together, as desired. Consume freely, room temperature or cooler.

• Pay particular attention to **carotene-rich foods** if flooding is part of your journey through menopause. Foods such as nettles, liquid chlorophyll, and carrots help you maintain energy when there is large blood loss; they are critical to the formation of healthy new blood. (See Appendix I.)

*Step 4. Sedate/Stimulate . . .*

• Press very firmly on either of these **acupressure points** for one minute out of every fifteen as an emergency sedative for flooding. One is located above the center of the upper lip (and under the nose). The other is right at the top of the head.

★ Fresh **shepherd's purse** (*Capsella bursa-pastoris*) herb, including seed pods and flowers, is a renowned remedy for women hemorrhaging from the uterus. Drink the tea freely; sip at least a cupful of the infusion daily. Use the tincture by the dropperful; put tincture under the tongue if the flooding is severe. With menopausal flooding, expect to see some result within a few hours, and strong results in a day or two. If not, try a dropperful of blue cohosh (*Caulophyllum thralictroides*) or trillium (*Trillium species*) root tincture up to 4 times a day for several days. Women with fibroids may need to continue daily use of shepherd's purse for months.

★ **Witch hazel** (*Hamamelis virginiana*) bark/leaf infusion or tincture is my favorite for checking flooding. Unlike shepherd's purse, which contracts and shuts down the uterus, witch hazel allows normal menstruation. It also has a tonic effect on the uterus. Drink 1-3 cups/up to ¾ liter of the infusion daily. Take the tincture of the fresh bark by the dropperful. Bleeding will remain steady or diminish within a few hours and slow to nearer normal within two days if this herb is effective for you.

• Avoid blood-thinning herbs such as red clover (*Trifolium pratense*), alfalfa (*Medicago sativa*), cleavers (*Galium aparine*), pennyroyal

(*Hedeoma pulegioides*), willow bark (*Salix*), and wintergreen (*Galtheria procumbens*). Thin blood is more likely to hemorrhage.

★ **Acupuncture** treatments are extremely helpful for women with severe menopausal flooding. Daily treatments during the flooding commonly stop acute blood loss. Frequent treatments during the luteal phase help prevent further flooding.

• Sip **cinnamon** infusion or take 5-10 drops tincture every fifteen minutes, to slow flooding and relieve uterine cramping. CAUTION: Do not use cinnamon oil.

***Step 5a. Use supplements . . .***

★ Use essential fatty acids (EFAs) to sedate flooding. Try 4-8 capsules or 1-2 tablespoons/15-30 ml daily of oils of flax seed, borage seed, black currant seed, or evening primrose seed; they provide a powerful supplement to natural prostaglandin production. Try this for at least six weeks.

• Supplements of zinc, copper, and iodine have been used to diminish flooding. CAUTION: Overdoses are toxic.

• Vitamin $B_6$, 25-50 mg daily, can help assimilation of iron and thus minimize anemia from flooding, and, in some cases, reduce flooding. CAUTION: More than 100 mg $B_6$ taken daily for more than 6 months can be toxic. (See Appendix I for herbal sources.)

★ Avoid aspirin, Midol, and large doses of ascorbic acid (vitamin C supplements) as they thin blood and may increase bleeding.

***Step 5b. Use drugs . . .***

• **Progestin** (synthetic progesterone) taken during the luteal phase, or an injection of Depo-Provera, are alternatives to surgery for women with uncontrollable, life-threatening flooding.

***Step 6. Break and enter . . .***

★ Flooding is frequently caused by IUDs (intra-uterine devices inserted for birth control). If you have one, now's the time to have it removed. (See Birth Control, page 38.)

• Surgical remedies for flooding involve dilating the cervix and inserting an instrument to remove the blood-rich lining from the womb. In many instances, the flooding ceases and menopause continues uneventfully.

☞ **Aspiration curettage**, like a clinical abortion, removes a thin layer of the endometrium. It can be done under local anesthetic and without a hospital stay. This procedure is far less risky to you and your uterus than the more common D&C. Tests for cancer can easily be done on the aspirated material if need be. The endometrium regrows naturally.

☞ **D&C** (dilation and curettage) is the standard modern medical treatment for women with menstrual hemorrhage. In a D&C a layer of the endometrium is scraped away. This is done under general anesthetic and requires a hospital stay. The endometrium regrows.

☞ **TCRE** (trans-cervical resection of the endometrium) completely removes the endometrium. It rarely regrows. This may be done under local anesthesia. Over 90 percent of 234 women who chose this treatment rather than a hysterectomy reported relief from their heavy bleeding. The long-term results of TCRE are unknown, as it is a fairly new procedure.

• More than 25 percent of all hysterectomies are done to control flooding. Menopausal flooding doesn't last forever; hysterectomy does.

★ Note: Many women use 30-60 drops of **echinacea** tincture several times daily for the week preceding and the several weeks following any surgery to strengthen and nourish the immune system and help prevent infection.

# Fibroids

*"My fibroid was the size of a twelve-week pregnancy, or so I was told. When I asked my uterus what was up, it replied: 'If you aren't going to take steps to get pregnant, I will.' Discovering that there was a shared desire, I realigned with my uterus and now my fibroid comes and goes but has never again grown so large."*

**Step 1. Collect information . . .**

Uterine fibroid tumors are non-malignant growths in smooth muscle tissue. They occur so frequently (in up to half of all women over forty) that they may be considered normal. Women of color are three times as likely to have fibroids as white women.

The occasional fibroid can reach the size of a grapefruit or even a cantaloupe (medical literature reports an 80 pound/35 kilo fibroid!), but the majority of fibroids remain marble-sized or smaller and cause no discomfort or distress. Fibroids may temporarily enlarge during the menopausal years.

If you have no symptoms, but are told during a routine pelvic exam that you have fibroid tumors, don't worry. You don't have cancer. (Tumor means a swelling or growth; most tumors are benign. Less than 0.1% of all fibroids are malignant.)

Small fibroids are fairly easy to resolve. As they cause no symptoms — and often disappear spontaneously — they need cause you no concern. Larger fibroids will contribute to menopausal flooding and other complaints. Large fibroids are more difficult to resolve, but often slowly shrink with treatment. Very large fibroids can exert pressure on the bladder, bowels, or sensitive pelvic nerves, causing a variety of symptoms including pelvic pain, frequent urination, constipation, low back pain, irritable bowels, and severe menstrual/menopausal flooding.

Fibroids are hormone dependent. They disappear after menopause except in women who take supplemental hormones (estrogen replacement). Treatment of fibroids is the most frequently cited reason for hysterectomy.

### Step 2. Engage the energy . . .

• **Reiki** treatments have been helpful to some women with large fibroids.

• Many healers perceive fibroids as energy "stuck" in the uterus. To begin to move this energy: Sit or recline comfortably and draw your attention to your breath. Imagine that you are breathing out of your womb and then out of your vagina. Pause a moment. Breathe into your vagina and into your womb. Pause a moment and feel the breath spiral inside the uterus. Breathe out. Continue for at least ten breaths.

• Supportive therapy can help expose and move emotional energies which our culture encourages us to stuff in our bodies.

### Step 3. Nourish and tonify . . .

• One woman's fibroids (and menstrual cramps) disappeared within three months of beginning a vigorous **exercise** program.

★ **Lignins**, found in all whole grains, are anti-estrogenic. As fibroids seem to be estrogen/progesterone dependent (they increase in size during pregnancy when these hormones are highest and disappear after menopause, when these hormones are lowest), it is possible that consuming three or more servings of whole grains daily could offer prevention or cure. Lignins are present in decreasing order in: flax seed, rye, buckwheat, millet, soya, oats, barley, corn, rice, and wheat.

• The glycerine macerate of *Sequoia gigantica* buds is recommended by Swiss herbalist Rina Nissim for women dealing with uterine fibroids. Use 50 drops, 1-3 times daily, in a small glass of water.

★ Rina Nissim also suggests an **anti-estrogenic brew** for women with fibroids. It contains equal parts tinctures of: black currant buds or leaves (*Ribes nigrum*), gromwell herb or seeds (*Lithospermum offici-*

*nalis*), lady's mantle herb (*Alchemilla vulgaris*), chaste tree berries (*Vitex agnus-castus*), yarrow flowers (*Achillea millefolium*), and wild pansy flowers (*Viola tricolor*). Dosage: a teaspoonful/5 ml upon arising. Expect noticeable results with 2-4 months. This is such a beautifully conceived formula, that, like a superb soup recipe, any ingredients may be omitted without destroying the integrity of the whole. In fact, any one of these herbs — used as a simple — would be extremely beneficial to a pre-menopausal woman dealing with fibroids.

★ **Vitex** berry tincture, 25-30 drops taken twice daily, may shrink small fibroids within two months, but don't hesitate to use it for up to two years.

• Ask someone to burn **moxa** over the area of the fibroid while you envision the heat releasing the treasures in your uterus. What is locked up in this fibroid? What can you give birth to? (It's OK to birth a monster.) Do this 4-6 times a week for at least six weeks.

### Step 4. Sedate/Stimulate . . .

★ **Acupuncture** treatments can shrink fibroids.

★ **Cotton root bark** (*Gossypium*), primarily known as an extremely effective abortifacient, is a specific agent for stopping flooding due to fibroids. Use ½ cup/125 ml of infusion every half hour as needed, or a dropperful of the tincture every 5-10 minutes until hemorrhage stops.

• Try warm **castor oil** packs over the fibroid; or try compressing with a towel soaked in hot **ginger water**.

★ CAUTION: Dong Quai/Dang Gui can easily increase size of fibroids. Limit use to no more than 10 drops daily or avoid totally.

### Step 5b. Use drugs . . .

• Hormone replacement (ERT/HRT) encourages the growth of fibroids.

• When bleeding from fibroids is excessive and threatening, an injection of Depo-Provera can be used to stop the bleeding, thus gaining time for the slower-acting natural remedies to take effect.

### Step 6. Break and enter . . .

• When only the fibroid is removed, the procedure is called **myomectomy**. This surgery saves the uterus but requires a talented and sensitive surgeon. Extensive bleeding during surgery is the norm. The fibroids may regrow. The use of laser myomectomy reduces the large blood loss associated with removal of fibroids.

• **Hysterectomy** is the modern Western remedy for fibroids. While removal of the uterus may save the life of a woman who is in danger of hemorrhaging severely from a large fibroid, the mere presence of fibroids is not sufficient reason to consider a hysterectomy.

So frequently are women advised to have their uteruses removed, often for no better reason than fibroids felt during a routine exam, that by the age of sixty more than one-third of all American women will have given up their wombs to the surgeons. Fully half of these women will experience loss of sexual desire, urinary problems, and severe, early menopause (even when the ovaries are retained). Adhesions frequently form on the intestines after a hysterectomy and can cause emergency surgery and/or death.

• If you choose surgery to remedy your fibroids, use these remedies as well to protect your health and speed healing from the operation:

☞ Use 25 drops of echinacea root tincture 1-3 times a day, for three days before the operation and seven to ten days after.

☞ Try acupuncture treatments, before and after surgery.

☞ Avoid blood-borne diseases by donating some of your own blood to be used during the surgery.

☞ One woman created a ritual for "giving my uterus away rather than giving up on my uterus."

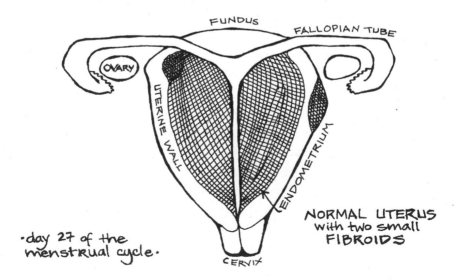

FUNDUS

FALLOPIAN TUBE

OVARY

UTERINE WALL

ENDOMETRIUM

·day 27 of the menstrual cycle·

NORMAL UTERUS with two small FIBROIDS

CERVIX

# Spotting

*"I used to feel a little twinge of pain when I would ovulate. Then one month there was a spot of fresh blood. This has gradually increased, and now I spot for several days around ovulation."*

### Step 1. Collect information . . .

Vaginal bleeding other than a menstrual flow is called spotting. The amount of blood may be barely enough to stain the underwear or it may be enough to require a minipad.

Like flooding, spotting and staining are normal manifestations of menopause, as well as indicators of possible reproductive distress.

Causes of spotting include menopause, ovulation, unsuspected miscarriage or spontaneous abortion, cervical infections, polyps, cervical dysplasia, irritation or infection from an IUD, cancer, and hyperplasia.

**Seek help if more than two years have passed since your last period and you begin to spot or stain. Also seek help if your staining continues for more than ten days.**

### Step 2. Engage the energy . . .

• There are two primary homeopathic remedies for women with menopausal spotting: *China* is for the woman who also floods, feels weak, and is often depressed. *Pulsatilla* is for the woman who is highly emotional.

### Step 3. Nourish and tonify . . .

★ **Red raspberry leaf** is the ally of choice for the menopausal woman who is spotting for no known reason. Try at least 2 cups/500 ml of the infusion daily. Add some mint to lighten the taste, if you wish.

• **Ginger root** tea warms and nourishes the entire pelvis. Try a cup/250 ml a day, sweetened with honey, for several weeks. Regular menses may be re-established, or the spotting may temporarily increase, then stop.

### Step 4. Sedate/Stimulate . . .

• Cinnamon is a specific remedy for spotting. (See page 10.)

★ **Wild yam** root tincture (10-15 drops) or a full cup of tea can prevent and halt mid-cycle spotting by contributing to progesterone production. So can **chaste tree.**

### Step 5b. Use drugs . . .

• Birth control pills may be prescribed to control spotting. This is not advised for women older than forty.

• A progesterone challenge — ten days of synthetic hormone — is another remedy suggested for troubling spotting. (See list of herbs rich in progesterone precursors, page 44.)

**Step 6. Break and enter . . .**

• Endometrial biopsy and D&C are used to diagnose and cure spotting. Support your healing from these surgeries with echinacea tincture. (See page 14.)

# Menstrual Cramps

*"The hot flashes didn't slow me down, but the menstrual cramps did. I remember cramps like this when I was a teen. I vaguely remember hot water bottles, my mother's tender touch, thick novels, time alone to dream, to envision how my life would flower."*

**Step 1. Collect information . . .**

The amount and intensity of your menstrual cramping may very well change during your **Change**. The major problem menopausal women face in dealing with cramps is that most herbs and many drugs which relieve cramping also increase flooding. Here are some that don't (note exceptions).

**Step 2. Engage the energy . . .**

• Menstrual cramps remind us to take time alone.

• Sit in a hot bath and flow, melt, dissolve, relax, release, let go.

**Step 3. Nourish and tonify . . .**

★ **Liferoot** is the remedy for women with intense cramps, even when accompanied by severe fatigue, nausea, and faintness. Try 5-10 drops of fresh flower tincture daily during your luteal phase for at least three months before expecting full relief.

★ The viburnums, **black haw** and **cramp bark**, are superb allies for the menopausal woman who is cramping and flooding. They provide astringent action, powerful antispasmodic effects, and a rich supply of hormonal precursors. Use 10-20 drops of the tincture as often as needed.

• **Garden sage** tea is hormone-rich and astringent, and, like all mints, a remedy for menstrual cramps. Most other mints, however (such as catnip, a common and highly effective remedy for cramps), increase flooding, and are best avoided.

**Step 4. Sedate/Stimulate . . .**

• If you aren't flooding, and don't think you will, use **ginger** tea (from fresh or dried roots) to ease your menstrual cramps.

• A dose of 5-15 drops of **motherwort** tincture generally eliminates menstrual cramps promptly; it may provoke flooding, however.

★ **Valerian** root tincture, 30 drops repeated as needed, eases menstrual pain dramatically. Valerian makes many women sleepy and a few hyperactive.

**Step 5b. Use drugs . . .**

• Aspirin eases menstrual cramps but can provoke flooding. So can Midol. Willow bark (*Salix*) tincture is as effective as aspirin in relieving cramps but less likely to cause flooding. Best in vinegar.

**Step 6. Break and enter . . .**

★ A Crone's Year Away will disrupt every part of your life, breaking down carefully established patterns. It's time for **Change**.

# Cessation of Menses

*"I was bleeding when the news came that he had been killed. I stopped within the hour and haven't had a period since. I was 38 then; I'm 62 now."*

**Step 1. Collect information . . .**

Lack of menstrual flow (indicating, usually, lack of ovulation as well) is called amenorrhea. Amenorrhea is common off and on during the menopausal years until it becomes the permanent state of the Crone. Menopausal amenorrhea needs no remedy.

Amenorrhea not associated with menopause is a serious problem, however. Bone loss during one premenopausal month without menses is the equivalent of one year's bone loss post-menopausally. The most common reasons for the menses to disappear before menopause (excluding pregnancy) are lack of body fat (from eating disorders or heavy athletic training) and stress. The following remedies are for women who believe their amenorrhea is not related to menopause.

**Step 2. Engage the energy . . .**

• If the stress is related to loss/grief, try homeopathic *Ignatia*.

• If the menses stop after a severe emotional shock, try the tissue salt *Natrum mur.*

### Step 3. Nourish and tonify . . .

★ **Nettle** leaf infusion has reportedly returned the monthly flow to women drinking it regularly, even in their sixties!

• If the menses have stopped due to lack of body fat, use the remedies for **weight gain**, page 152.

• If emotional upheaval has stopped your menstrual cycles, seek **supportive counseling** or a therapy group to help you work with your grief, anger, and repressed memories.

★ **Dong Quai/Dang Gui** is frequently the remedy of choice for unexplained cessation of menses. She nourishes the "palace of the child" and establishes regular cycles. CAUTION: Avoid if you are prone to flooding, or have fibroids.

### Step 4. Stimulate/Sedate . . .

• **Acupuncture** treatments can be quite useful in re-establishing normal menstrual/hormonal cycling.

• Try strong **pennyroyal** (*Hedeoma pulegioides* or *Mentha pulegium*) tea, a cupful/250 ml or more a day, for the three days of the new moon, to stimulate menstrual bleeding and restore regular cycling.

### Step 5a. Use supplements . . .

• Supplements of **vitamin E**, 200-600 IU daily, have helped women restore ovulation and menstruation. Consistent use brings best results.

### Step 6. Break and enter . . .

• Ten or more sessions of Rolfing (body work focused on breaking patterns held in the fascia between the muscles) can restore menstrual cycles for women not yet in the menopausal years.

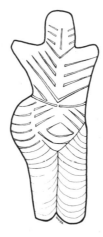

# Preventing Osteoporosis

*"It is a bone-deep change you are going to experience, my beloved,"
counsels Grandmother Growth. "You must open to your very marrow
for this transformation. No cell is to remain untouched. You are to open
more than you ever dreamed you could open, more than you have opened
in birth or in passion. You open now to the breath of mortality as it
plays the bone flute of your being. What can you do but dance to the
haunting melody, develop a passion for an elegant posture and a long
stride?*

*Ah, yes," Grandmother Growth smiles rather wantonly, "it would
do you well to develop a taste for dark greens tarted with vinegar and
mated with garlic. These things will build a fine bone to support you as
you become Crone."*

Did you know that your bones are always changing? Every day of
your life, bone cells die and new bone cells are created. Until the age
of 25-35, you can easily make lots of bone cells. After you replace the
ones that die, you lengthen your bones (i.e., grow) and lay down bone
mass with surplus cells.

As you age, however, it becomes harder to make bone cells. When
more bone cells die than you create, osteoporosis has begun. By the
age of forty it is likely that you have begun to lose bone mass. You've
only lost a little if you exercise and eat calcium-rich foods regularly.
You may have lost quite a bit if you sit a lot and regularly consume foods
that interfere with calcium absorption (such as coffee, soda pop, alcohol,
white flour products, processed meats, nutritional yeast, and bran).

No matter what your lifestyle choices, bone mass decreases during
the menopausal years. For about five years right after the last menses,
the bones apparently reject calcium and osteoporosis increases, giving
rise to the belief that ERT, taken as soon as menopause begins and
continued for several decades, is the only hope for women who want
to avoid broken bones and a bed-ridden old age. But bones start
absorbing calcium once again when this "bone-pause" is past. And
consumption of calcium-rich plants, combined with moderate exercise,
can reverse osteoporosis. And women who faithfully take ERT still
experience bone changes and spinal crush fractures.

Doesn't ERT increase bone density, though? Yes, but dense bone mass does not guarantee freedom from fracture. Bones that resist breaking are flexible. The dense bones of women taking calcium supplements and ERT are often rigid. Flexible bone mass is built with balanced mineral intake (leafy greens, herbal infusions) and exercise.

When you take ERT, bone cell creation is not improved. Bone cell death is slowed down, suppressed. Unfortunately, there is a rebound effect, and the rate of bone loss can increase greatly if you stop taking ERT. When you build bones with green allies and exercise, bone cell creation is stimulated and supported. If you must eat poorly or miss your physical activity for some weeks, bone mass is still retained.

ERT, taken as menopause begins and continued for the rest of your life, might reduce your rate of post-menopausal fractures by as much as 40-60 percent. Frequent walks (you don't even have to sweat) and a diet high in calcium-rich green allies (at least 1500 mg daily) consistently reduce post-menopausal fractures by at least 50 percent.

So long as you take ERT, you will have to pay drug bills and submit to invasive check-ups to rule out reproductive cancers. With green allies and exercise, you have no drug costs and no increased risk of cancer.

It is never too late to build dense flexible bones, and it is never too soon. In fact, your best insurance for a fracture-free, strong-boned cronehood is to **build bone mass before menopause**. The more exercise and calcium you get in your younger years, the more ultimate benefit you'll reap. The more bone mass you have by age 40, the more you'll have at 55, when you are crowned Crone, and the more you'll have at 75, when it really counts.

---

**The most important factors in developing and maintaining bone mass from puberty to menopause are:**

◇ sufficient dietary calcium
◇ adequate loading onto the skeleton (exercise)
◇ uninterrupted reproductive status (no loss of menses due to low weight)

---

*"A woman has lost half of all the spongy bone (spine, wrist) she'll ever lose by the age of 50, but very little of the dense (hip, hand, forearm) bone. Attention to bone formation at every stage of life is vital; there is no time when you are too old to create healthy new bone."*   —Advice from an American MD

# Calcium

*Step 1. Collect information . . .*

Calcium is, without a doubt, the most important mineral in your body. In fact, calcium makes up more than half of the total mineral content of your body. Calcium is crucial to the regular beating of your heart, your metabolism, the functioning of your muscles, the flow of impulses along your nerves, the regulation of your cellular membranes, the strength of your bones, the health of your teeth and gums, and your vital blood-clotting mechanisms. Calcium is so critical to your life that you have a gland (the parathyroid) that does little else than monitor blood levels of calcium and secrete hormones to insure optimum levels of calcium at all times.

When you consume more calcium than you use, you are in a positive calcium balance: extra usable calcium is stored in the bones and you gain bone mass (insoluble or unusable calcium may be excreted, or stored in soft tissue, or deposited at the joints). When you consume less calcium than you use, you are in a negative calcium balance: the parathyroid produces a hormone that releases calcium stores from the bone, and you lose bone mass.

To insure a positive calcium balance, avoid arthritis, prevent kidney stones, and create dense, flexible bones for your menopausal journey, take care during your premenopausal years to:

☞ **Eat three or more calcium-rich foods daily.**

☞ **Avoid those foods and habits that use up large amounts of calcium.**

☞ **Include synergistic foods that magnify the effectiveness of calcium.**

☞ **Avoid calcium supplements taken as a matter of course.**

*Step 2. Engage the energy . . .*

• Homeopathic tissue salts, especially *Silica*, are recommended for improving the health of bones.

• What does it mean to you to support yourself? To be supported? To stand on your own? To have backbone in your life?

*Step 3. Nourish and tonify . . .*

★ To mimimize osteoporosis, eat three or more calcium-rich foods daily and improve calcium utilization with synergistic foods. (See boxes, pages 23-25.)

★ **Horsetail** herb (*Equisetum arvense*) works like a charm for those premenopausal women who have already begun to experience periodontal bone loss or difficulty with fracture healing. Taken as a tea, once or twice a day, spring-gathered horsetail herb dramatically increases healing and strength in bones. CAUTION: Horsetail gathered after the first spring growth may be overly abundant in silica, irritating the kidneys and sensitizing the nerves.

### Step 4. Stimulate/Sedate . . .

• Calcium requires an acid environment for maximum digestibility. **Increase hydrochloric acid** production for digestion of calcium, iron, and other nutrients.

☞ Drink **lemon juice** in water with or after your meal.

☞ Take 10-15 drops **dandelion** root tincture in several ounces/50-60 ml of water about fifteen minutes before you eat.

☞ Add 2 tablespoons/30 ml apple cider **vinegar** and 2 tablespoons/ 30 ml raw honey or blackstrap **molasses** to a cup/250 ml of hot water; drink with or after your meal.

☞ Use calcium-rich herbal vinegars in your salad dressing.

• Coffee, white sugar, tobacco, alcohol, fiber pills, bran, nutritional yeast, and greens rich in oxalic acid bind calcium, rendering it unusable by the body. Meat, salt, fluoride, and phosphorus-rich foods such as soda pop and white flour products use up calcium stores in the bones. If taken or eaten on a daily basis, singly or together, these things contribute substantially to osteoporosis. (See following.)

• The digestion of protein produces acids which are buffered with calcium when excreted in the urine. Thus foods rich in protein but low in calcium (such as red meat) result in calcium loss from the bones. Use high-calcium protein sources instead: **tahini, tofu, oats, seaweed, sardines, salmon, yogurt, oatmeal, nettles, dandelion leaves.** (Not all tofu contains calcium; check the label.) NOTE: The highest incidence of osteoporosis is found in countries (USA and Scandinavia, for example) where the consumption of dairy products and meat is the highest.

• **Excess salt** in the diet produces a urine loaded with calcium. Women eating 3900 mg sodium daily excreted 30 percent more calcium than those eating 1600 mg daily (British Medical Journal 299, 1989). Table salt is rarely the problem; the main sources of dietary sodium are processed and canned foods. Do not attempt to eliminate salt entirely from your diet; it is necessary for health. Seaweed is an excellent calcium-rich source of salt.

• **Excess phosphorus** accelerates bone loss and demineralization. Phosphorus compounds are second only to salt as food additives. For strong bones, use sparingly or not at all: soda pop; white flour products, especially if "enriched" (bagels, cookies, cakes, donuts, pasta, bread); preserved meats (bacon, ham, sausage, lunch meat, and hot dogs);

supermarket breakfast cereals; canned fruit; processed potato products such as frozen fries and instant mashed potatoes; processed cheeses; instant soups and puddings.

• Some greens contain **oxalic acid**, which loves to change into calcium oxalate, thus inhibiting calcium absorption from these greens. This isn't to say that you should never eat spinach, swiss chard (silver beet), beet greens, wood sorrel, or rhubarb, just that you shouldn't consider them calcium sources. Consider them iron sources.

## Improve Calcium Utilization with Synergistic Foods

◇ Calcium and **vitamin D** work together. Alfalfa and nettle contain both. Use either as an infusion. Or eat more salmon, halibut, mackerel, and free-range eggs. Or get 20 minutes of sun daily.

◇ **Vitamin K** is crucial to calcium use. Good sources are potatoes, yogurt, molasses, leafy greens, green tea, kelp, and nettles.

◇ **Magnesium** is another co-worker with calcium. Note that the calcium-rich herbs are usually magnesium-rich as well, especially oatstraw, kelp, nettle, horsetail, and sage.

◇ The mineral **boron** has an effect on rate of bone formation, both as a synergist with calcium and as a nourisher to hormone production. Increasing levels of boron in the diet increases blood levels of estrogen and progesterone. In one study, blood levels of estrogen in post-menopausal women taking boron supplements began to rise within a week, and were equivalent within the month to those of women on ERT. Organic fruits and vegetables are the best sources of boron.

◇ See Appendix I for further herbal sources of these vitamins and minerals.

◇ **Lactose** and other natural sugars boost calcium absorption.

★ **Phosphorus** helps calcium unless you overdo it, and that, sadly, is very easy to do. Virtually all processed foods and carbonated drinks contain bone-robbing amounts of phosphorus. Follow these rules to avoid phosphorus overload and improve calcium absorption:

   ☞ **Drink water or herbal infusions instead of soda pop.**
   ☞ **Eat only whole grain breads, noodles, cookies, crackers.**
   ☞ **Replace meat with beans or fish for most meals.**
   ☞ **Rely on fresh foods rather than preserved, processed ones.**

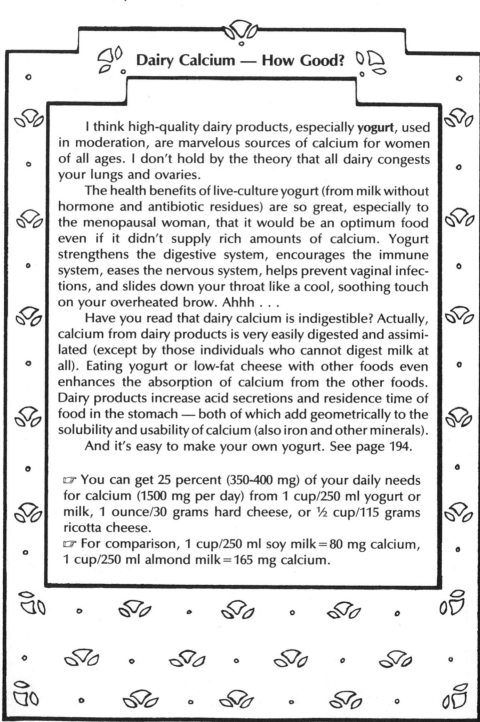

## Dairy Calcium — How Good?

I think high-quality dairy products, especially **yogurt**, used in moderation, are marvelous sources of calcium for women of all ages. I don't hold by the theory that all dairy congests your lungs and ovaries.

The health benefits of live-culture yogurt (from milk without hormone and antibiotic residues) are so great, especially to the menopausal woman, that it would be an optimum food even if it didn't supply rich amounts of calcium. Yogurt strengthens the digestive system, encourages the immune system, eases the nervous system, helps prevent vaginal infections, and slides down your throat like a cool, soothing touch on your overheated brow. Ahhh . . .

Have you read that dairy calcium is indigestible? Actually, calcium from dairy products is very easily digested and assimilated (except by those individuals who cannot digest milk at all). Eating yogurt or low-fat cheese with other foods even enhances the absorption of calcium from the other foods. Dairy products increase acid secretions and residence time of food in the stomach — both of which add geometrically to the solubility and usability of calcium (also iron and other minerals).

And it's easy to make your own yogurt. See page 194.

☞ You can get 25 percent (350-400 mg) of your daily needs for calcium (1500 mg per day) from 1 cup/250 ml yogurt or milk, 1 ounce/30 grams hard cheese, or ½ cup/115 grams ricotta cheese.

☞ For comparison, 1 cup/250 ml soy milk=80 mg calcium, 1 cup/250 ml almond milk=165 mg calcium.

# ◌◌ Eat Three or More Calcium-Rich Foods Daily ◌◌

◊ **Calcium-rich herbs** include nettle, sage, chickweed, red clover, comfrey leaf, raspberry leaf, and oatstraw. Enjoy a tasty infusion of any one every day. Count a big mug of infusion as 250-300 mg calcium. Add a big pinch of horsetail to your brew and increase the calcium by 10 percent.

◊ **Cooked greens** provide abundant, highly usable calcium. One cup/250 ml of cooked broccoli, kale, turnip greens, or mustard greens contains about 200 mg calcium. One cup/250 ml of cooked collards, wild onions, lamb's quarter, or amaranth greens, about 400 mg calcium.

◊ Slurp up at least a tablespoon/15 ml of "Old Sour Puss Mineral Mix" (page 192) daily; it supplies 200-300 mg calcium. (Or 350-400 mg if you add a tablespoon/15 ml of blackstrap molasses.)

◊ **Dried fruit** is a fairly good place to look for calcium. There's 65 mg in 3 small figs, a handful of raisins, 4 dates, or 8 prunes. Soak some for breakfast tomorrow, or try "Fruit Fix," page 189.

◊ Because they are made with lime, which is a form of calcium, **corn tortillas** are an excellent calcium source. Two supply 120 mg.

◊ See recipe for "Strong Bones Stew," page 189.

◊ See recipe for "Bonny Bony Brew," page 190.

◊ Menopausal women do best when eating 1500 mg or more of calcium daily.

• Although chocolate also contains oxalic acid, the levels are so low as to have only a negligible effect on calcium metabolism. An ounce/3000 mg of chocolate will bind 15-20 mg of calcium, while an ounce of cooked spinach will bind 100-125 mg calcium. Bittersweet (dark) chocolate is a source of iron. As with any stimulant, daily use of chocolate is certainly not advised. My personal experience has been that chocolate is an important and helpful ally for women and our guilt about occasional use (even in large quantity) is damaging to our ability to hear and respond to our body wisdom. My advice, in brief, is this: if you have a sudden urge to eat chocolate — do it. If you want to eat chocolate every day — eat more weeds instead.

### Step 5a. Use supplements . . .

• Calcium-fortified orange juice is the only way to get a form of supplemental calcium (calcium citrate maleate) that is remarkably easy to digest and absorb. If you must supplement, do it this way. Crumbly tablets of calcium citrate are a close second best.

• Calcium gluconate, calcium lactate, and calcium carbonate (if chewable) are acceptable sources of supplemental calcium. Up to 1500 mg daily may be taken. Do not use dolomite, bone meal, or oyster shell, as they generally contain an abundance of lead and other undesirable minerals.

• For even better bones, take 500 mg magnesium (not citrate) with your calcium. Better yet, wash your calcium pill down with a glass of herbal infusion; that will provide not only magnesium but lots of other synergistic minerals, too.

• Calcium supplements are more effective in divided doses. Two doses of 250 mg, taken morning and night, actually provide more usable calcium than a 1000 mg tablet.

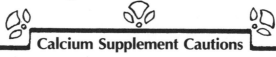

## Calcium Supplement Cautions

◇ Calcium supplements increase bacterial adherence in the bladder and urinary tract, thus increasing the likelihood of urinary tract infections and cystitis.

◇ Kidney stones may be precipitated by taking daily doses of calcium supplements that exceed 2500 mg, and drinking too little water.

◇ There is much folklore, and even some slight scientific evidence, linking arthritis to use of calcium supplements.

### Step 5b. Use drugs . . .

• If you are currently taking ERT or HRT in hopes of preventing osteo-porosis, you can also safely use any of the above remedies. If you wish, you can gradually cut back on your hormone dose by shaving your daily pills smaller and smaller, as you increase your intake of hormone- and calcium-rich foods/herbs.

### Step 6. Break and enter . . .

• Hi-tech tests of bone density are expensive and meaningless unless you are prepared to take ERT, says the AMA. (See page 163.)

# Weight Gain

*"Pack your bags for the journey," Grandmother Growth advises softly. "Your Change may be rough in places, so cushion yourself. Your Change may have some hard edges, so let your contours round. Your wise blood is stirring and you are learning to let it move without attaching fear to its meanderings. In the same way, you can allow with grace your natural weight gain. Struggling with your weight or dieting is bad medicine for you now, resulting only in thin bones that break easily, extreme hormone shifts that will keep you from sleeping and thinking, and an inner fire reduced to ashes or burning out of control. Pack your bags, slowly, dear one. There is no rush," sighs Grandmother Growth, closing her eyes and sinking into a nap.*

The best ally you can have on your menopausal journey is ten "extra" pounds. I know you don't want to hear this. I understand how difficult it is to desire ten extra pounds (or accept it happening to you, as it does to most menopausal women). You may have spent much of your life trying to get rid of ten extra pounds. The American male-dominant culture's insistence on "beauty equals thin" makes the diet industry a tremendous money-maker in America. When thin and young is the standard of beauty, the menopausal woman finds it difficult to maintain a positive self image as she sees herself transforming into a thick-waisted, silver-haired Crone.

Nonetheless, repeat to yourself: "The best ally I can have on my menopausal journey is ten 'extra' pounds."

I am not talking about ten pounds of pure fat. You want ten pounds of fat supported by muscle and bone. And you want to gain that ten pounds very, very slowly; ideally, about a pound a year after the age of forty, so you'll be "in shape" for the intense part of your menopausal journey around the age of fifty.

### Step 1. Collect information . . .

• Fat cells make estrogen. Weighty women have a later menopause, less severe hot flashes, a more gradual **Change**, and denser bones (less osteoporosis). Thinner women have a harder journey through menopause.

### Step 2. Engage the energy . . .

• Give yourself permission to **take up more space**. Allow your needs to be uppermost. Enlarge your view of yourself. Enlarge your world.

• If you don't already do an hour or more of yoga, tai chi, or some other **meditative physical activity** weekly, begin . . . now.

• Go to an art gallery, or get a book from your library, and find a picture of a beautiful naked woman with a proud belly. Meditate on/with her.

### Step 3. Nourish and tonify . . .

★ The best way to slowly gain ten pounds of hormone-ready fat, powerful muscles, and strong bones is to include one serving of a **high calorie hormone-rich food** and one serving of a **super mineral-rich food** in your diet every day.

☞ High-calorie, hormone-rich foods include homemade beer, hops tea, flax seed oil, wheat germ oil, alfalfa seeds (not sprouted), olives.

☞ Super mineral-rich foods include nettle infusion, cooked wild greens, oats and oatstraw infusion, seaweed, spirulina, whey, wheat grass, barley green, chickweed salad.

★ The addition of 2-3 beers a week (preferably home-brewed) to your diet will slowly increase your weight, improve your memory, soothe your nerves, and improve your immune system. A cup of hops tea with a spoonful of barley malt sweetener is a non-alcoholic alternative.

### Step 4. Sedate/Stimulate . . .

• SAD (seasonal affective disorder) is associated with intense cravings for starchy foods, overeating, and unwanted weight gain. See remedies for depression, pages 72-77.

• There are herbal remedies sold for weight loss that include diuretic and laxative herbs in sufficient quantity to disturb your electrolyte balance through excess fluid loss. This loss can be life threatening, especially during the menopausal years, when heart and adrenal functions are unstable. Avoid such combinations.

• If you are determined to lose weight during your menopausal years, here are three safe ways to proceed.

☞ Drink up to a quart/liter of fresh warm (not cold) soy milk as your breakfast. Otherwise, eat normally. (**Fresh soy milk** does not come in boxes. It can be made at home or purchased out of the dairy case at a health food store.)

☞ Gently simmer a handful of dried or fresh **bladderwrack (fucus) seaweed** for 15 minutes in enough water to cover. Strain and drink a cup or two (250-500 ml) a day for no more than three months.

☞ Eat a cup/250 ml of fresh **chickweed** daily or take a dropperful of the fresh plant tincture in some water during or after your meal.

### Step 5b. Use drugs . . .

• Appetite-suppressant drugs upset your metabolic rate and make it harder and harder for you to maintain a normal weight with a normal diet. Avoid all drugs and herbs that claim to suppress your hunger.

### Step 6. Break and enter . . .

• I hear some famous people are having the excess fat liposuctioned out of their derrières and then injected into their face to plump out their wrinkles.

# PMS Forever?

*"Counting days will not get you through this Change, my love," warns Grandmother Growth. "You are on the way to transformation; do not expect predictability. Do not become alarmed when you experience yourself in totally new ways. You are changing, getting ready for a new birth, getting ready to be initiated into the third stage of your life as woman. Your wise blood and your wise hormones are shifting in their courses. They may flood, wash away their usual routes, rearrange their known boundaries. Are you ready for the ride of your life?"*

Over the years you've gotten to know the changes you'll experience in the days just before bleeding begins. Water retention, sore breasts, constipation/diarrhea/gas, emotional uproar — the symptoms are different for every woman, but all disappear with the onset of menstruation. Have you considered what it will be like to have your premenstrual changes without the release of menstruation?

I don't have a bowel movement the day before I bleed. Will I be a constipated crone? Probably not. The thing about the **Change** is that it *is* a change. Even your premenstrual problems are likely to change.

A few quick remedies then, for premenopausal premenstrual distresses, the ones you know and the ones you might get to know.

# Water Retention

*"I tried everything to ease the swelling in my fingers and ankles. My daughter suggested nettle infusion, but I hated the taste of it. I finally froze some into ice cubes and put them in everything I drank and within a week my ankles were trim again."*

### Step 1. Collect information . . .

Fluid retention or bloat is a menopausal and premenstrual problem easily remedied. Note that a tendency toward water retention indicates a weakness in the adrenals/kidneys (and possibly heart).

### Step 2. Engage the energy . . .

• Listen to a recording of running water, or, better yet, sit beside a gurgling brook or a noisy river. Feel the waters inside you moving, flowing, sliding . . .

• Sleeping with a lavender dream pillow will help correct a tendency toward water retention.

### Step 3. Nourish and tonify . . .

★ My favorite herbal ally for help with water retention is **dandelion**.. Take 10-20 drops of the tincture of the spring-dug root with meals and watch the edema recede. Continue for as long as you like. Dandelion not only helps remove excess fluid from the cells, it nourishes and tones the kidneys (and adrenals) and liver, increases the digestibility of all food, and offers plant hormones to ease your **Change**.

★ Frequent use of **nettle** leaf infusion, a cup or more a day, rapidly relieves (and helps prevent further episodes of) water retention. Nettle is a superb nourisher of the kidneys and adrenals.

• Regular use of **Dong Quai/Dang Gui** root relieves bloat.

### Step 4. Stimulate/Sedate . . .

★ Take **less salt**.

• **Limit fluids** if you tend to bloat. The more fluids you drink, the harder the kidneys have to work, and the more tired they get. When they get very tired, fluid builds up in the cells. Optimally, drink at least a quart/liter of fluids daily.

• In order of increasing potency, these common foods stimulate release of held fluid: **asparagus, corn** (and corn silk tea), **grapes, cucumber, watermelon** (and tea from the seeds), parsley, celery, black tea, and coffee. The first five are also tonic; use freely. The last four are not; use more sparingly.

★ **Exercise** and **massage** stimulate strong movement of your fluids.

### Step 5a. Use supplements . . .

• Large doses of **ascorbic acid** (vitamin C) increase fluid output from the kidneys, but may stress the kidneys and increase the likelihood of water retention in the future.

### Step 5b. Use drugs . . .

• Chemical diuretics leach potassium, contributing to osteoporosis. Switch to nettle or dandelion for superb results, and lovely side effects like increased energy and better digestion.

### Step 6. Break and enter . . .

• Catheterization, short-term or in-dwelling, is used to relieve the bladder when you are unable to void on your own. Daily drinks of cranberry juice, blueberry juice, or uva ursi infusion help prevent bladder infections, a frequent side effect of this treatment.

## Sore Breasts

### Step 1. Collect information . . .

Breast tenderness premenstrually is often associated with water retention. Further discomfort may come in the form of benign lumps which enlarge as the time of menses approaches (and shrink afterward). These discomforts may increase in some women during their menopausal years. For others, menopause brings relief at last from chronically tender nipples and breasts.

### Step 2. Engage the energy . . .

• Meditate on your breasts when they feel ultra-sensitive. Sit quietly and follow your breath. As you breathe out, imagine air, or water, or energy, or milk flowing out of your breasts. With each breath out, let this nourishing, healing, moving energy flow out of your breasts and into the world. Feel your breasts relaxing as they pour out abundance with each breath. Finish by breathing in and opening your eyes.

### Step 3. Nourish and tonify . . .

• Hormone-rich herbs can be helpful allies when your breasts are tender and sore. Try 10-20 drops **black cohosh** tincture, or 20-40 drops **vitex** tincture, or 5-10 drops **liferoot** tincture twice a day for the two weeks preceding your bleeding. Chewing on a Dong Quai/Dang Qui root for those two weeks will help, too.

★ Women who consumed at least 1300 mg of calcium daily from dietary sources (greens, yogurt) had less breast tenderness.

### Step 4. Sedate/Stimulate . . . .

★ Use large **cabbage** leaves, steamed whole until soft, to compress swollen, sore breasts.

• Gently stroke **St. Joan's wort oil** onto your aching breasts. This oil penetrates the nerve endings and relieves pain.

• Try the remedies for water retention (page 30). Swollen, sore breasts may be engorged with excess fluid.

• Some women note that consumption of caffeine-rich foods such as coffee, colas, and black tea increases breast engorgement, lumps, and tenderness. If you eliminate these foods from your diet for six weeks and then reintroduce them, you'll be able to tell if this is true for you.

### Step 5a. Use supplements . . .

• Calcium and magnesium levels are often low in women who report painful breast tenderness.

• Vitamin B complex is another important nutrient believed to help relieve sore breasts.

### Step 5b. Use drugs . . .

• Low doses of the "Pill," taken in a regular cycle, may induce regular hormonal cycling and relieve persistent breast swelling/soreness.

• So may progesterone pills and injections.

### Step 6. Break and enter . . .

• Mammograms, if you are going to have them at all, are best avoided when your breasts are swollen and tender. The image won't be as clear and you will needlessly suffer painful treatment.

# Digestive Distresses

*Step 1. Collect information . . .*

Menopausal constipation and indigestion are generally due to the slowing of the gastrointestinal tract (estrogen is a gastrointestinal stimulant) and heavy demands on the liver.

Hormone levels affect digestion in general and the motility of the intestinal tract specifically. When your levels of estrogen and progesterone change (as they do throughout menopause, during pregnancy, and before menstruation and birth), your bowel patterns change, too.

Your liver is, among other things, a recycling center. The hormones you make each day are broken down by the liver when they are no longer needed and their "parts" become available for the production of other hormones. During the menopausal years some hormones (such as LH and FSH) are produced in such enormous quantities that your liver may struggle to keep up with its recycling work, and have little energy left over for digestive duties.

*Step 2. Engage the energy . . .*

★ Before you eat, bless your food; say grace; thank the plants and animals who are giving away to nourish you; breathe in and feel grateful.

★ My mother's favorite way of preventing digestive distress and insuring regularity: eat at regular times and go to the toilet at regular times. You'd be surprised how effective this is.

• First thing in the morning, get yourself a cup of hot water (or herbal tea) and bring it back to bed. Sip it slowly, and gnaw gently on your bottom lip. Then lie on your back and bring your knees up, feet flat on the bed; place your palms on your belly and breathe deeply. As you feel you want to, rub (in spirals) up on the right, across the middle, and down on the left side of your abdomen. Soon you will feel the movement gathering momentum. Sit up slowly and head for the toilet.

*Step 3. Nourish and tonify . . .*

★ **Yellow dock root** vinegar or tincture is a wonderful ally for the woman with menopausual digestive distress. Daily doses of 1 teaspoonful/5 ml vinegar or 5-10 drops of tincture eliminate constipation, indigestion, and gas. Yellow dock is especially recommended for the woman who finds her early menopausal menses getting heavier.

★ **Dandelion** is everyone's favorite ally for a happy digestive system and liver. Use the leaves, rich in omega-3, in salads. Use the roots, rich in hormones, as a vinegar or tincture: take 1-2 teaspoons/5-10 ml vinegar or 10-20 drops tincture with meals. Dandelion helps relieve constipation, gas, indigestion, even gallstones.

★ Any kind of exercise, but especially walking, relieves digestive gas and improves transit time in the intestines. Oriental wisdom says the liver loves movement.

• Hormone-rich herbs are wonderful allies for dealing with menopausal digestive woes. Try a cup of **garden sage** tea.

• Motherwort, fenugreek, vitex, or black cohosh tinctures, taken daily, also strengthen digestion.

★ If constipation occurs due to a lessening of the moistening, lubricating cells in the colon, **slippery foods** such as slippery elm bark powder, oats, seaweed, flax seed, and seeds from *Plantago* (psyllium seeds if you buy them) are wonderfully helpful and relieving. I add a teaspoon/5 ml of each of the above to a cup/250 ml of rolled oats and 3 cups/750 ml of water and cook until thick.

★ **Acidophilus** liquid or powder relieves even chronic constipation. Use as much as you like.

### Step 4. Stimulate/Sedate . . .

• White flour products slow the digestive tract; so does meat. Whole grain products and lots of cooked greens will speed digestive flow.

• Add more **liquids** and **soft foods** to your diet — applesauce, yogurt, nourishing soups, herbal infusions — to help relieve constipation. Chew your food slowly and savor it. Drink sparingly at meals and lavishly between meals.

• Menopausal women will want to *avoid the use of bran* as a laxative in deference to building strong bones. Instead try **prunes** or prune juice, rhubarb with maple syrup, or **figs**. (See "Fruit Fix," page 189.)

★ My favorite remedy to relieve digestive and gas pain is **plain yogurt**. Sometimes even a tiny mouthful will bring instant relief. Acidophilus capsules work, too. So does **ginger** tea. Ahhh . . .

• Crushed hemp seed (*Cannabis sativa*) tea is used in several native pharmacopeias as an effective remedy for relieving menopausal constipation. Its full complement of amino acids and EFAs increase the benefit.

• Most so-called herbal laxatives are no better than drugs; they are addictive and destroy the tone of the intestinal peristaltic muscles. Except in rare cases (such as relief of constipation for a ninety-year-old woman confined to bed), I do not advise the use of aloes, senna, cascara sagrada, or combinations containing them.

*Step 5a. Use supplements . . .*

• Constipation and digestive distress is a common side effect of taking iron supplements. Try 5-10 drops of yellow dock root tincture daily instead.

*Step 6. Break and enter . . .*

• Enemas and colonics are last-resort techniques. They do not promote health and may strip the intestines of key fauna. Regular use of enemas is highly habit-forming.

## Emotional Uproar

*Step 1. Collect information . . .*

Raging and weeping are classic emotional manifestations of premenstrual, pregnant, and menopausal women. You may find your emotions harder to control as you enter your menopausal years. Men given hormone therapy against prostate cancer find themselves weeping in the midst of their daily routine!

*Step 2. Engage the energy . . .*

★ **Take time for yourself** when you find yourself weeping, yelling, raging, depressed, out of control. Create your own sacred space, even in a closet, where you can be alone, without responsibilities. You have a right to every one of your feelings.

• Begin (or deepen your commitment to working with) a **journal**. Use it to honor your feelings. Note how you care for yourself and your emotions. The **Change** is an opportunity to value your emotional self and to nourish all of your feelings, from grief to bliss, rage to outrageousness.

• Universal healing energy can help when your emotions are roaring. Channel it through your hands to your heart or womb; hold yourself.

*Step 3. Nourish and tonify . . .*

★ A cup of **garden sage** tea with honey will help restore your emotional center and soothe your irritated nerves. It is even said to cure insanity and hysteria. In Chinese herbal practice, honey is used (in tea, not cooked) to soften the energy of the liver when it is hardened by rage, frustration, and anger.

★ Pamper yourself. Get a **massage**. Cuddle with someone you love.

★ Mood swings are noticeably less dramatic when adequate dietary **calcium** nourishes your nerves and helps maintain even blood sugar levels.

• Slow-acting **liferoot** flower tincture, 5 drops, or slower-acting **vitex** berry tincture, 25-40 drops, taken daily for several weeks (especially premenstrually) will help you gradually unravel your emotional snarls.

• **Black cohosh** root tincture eases menopausal flashes and is said to cure hysteria, too. Try 10-20 drops once or twice a day for a month.

• Keep a **Dong Quai/Dang Gui** root handy to chew on when you feel like chewing someone's head off.

### Step 4. Sedate/Stimulate . . .

★ My remedy of choice for premenstrual emotional uproar is **mother-wort** — the calm, fierce-hearted motherwort, who helps you find your center in the wildest emotional storms. A dose of 5-15 drops can be taken at the time of upset; you'll feel calmer in a few minutes. Or take 10-20 drops twice a day for a month to help stabilize mood swings.

• **Valerian** root, used as a bath or taken as a tincture (15-20 drops as needed) is a powerful sleep-inducing sedative that also eases uterine cramps. Avoid long-term use.

### Step 5b. Use drugs . . .

• Mood-altering drugs, whether legal (tranquilizers, anti-depressants, alcohol) or illegal (cocaine, opium), easily lead to dependence.

### Step 6. Break and enter . . .

• Psychoactive plants (such as marijuana, psilocybin mushrooms, and mescaline), used in a safe setting, offer radically different results than mood-altering drugs. Psychoactive substances, used wisely, break open new neural pathways and establish easier flows of emotions and energy through both the physical and subtle bodies.

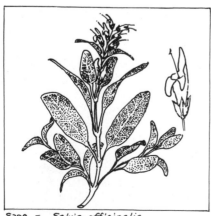

Sage — *Salvia officinalis*

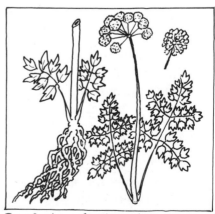

Dong Quai — *Angelica sinensis*

# Sore All Over

*Step 1. Collect information . . .*

This premenstrual distress seems to become more common during menopause. Muscles respond to the **Change** by feeling sore and cranky. Loss of sleep can also leave you feeling sore all over and lack of calcium can make your bones ache. I remember when they told me those aches in my legs were "growing pains." I guess they still are, only now I'm growing old.

*Step 2. Engage the energy . . .*

★ Homeopathic *Arnica* is an amazing remedy for sore and aching muscles.

★ Make a list of the things you are sore (upset, angry) about. Where do these things live in your body? With the help of an experienced bodyworker, loosen these sore places.

★ Go back to the Mother. Float in the ocean. Lie belly down on the earth. Naked. Let her ease you. Let her heal you.

★ Listen to a **relaxation** tape. Have someone show you how to do the yoga posture called the "Corpse Pose." Learn how to bring yourself to a deep state of inner quiet and peaceful mind.

*Step 3. Nourish and tonify . . .*

• Regular use of **Dong Quai/Dang Gui** is said to bring warmth and ease to achy, spasming muscles. Try 10-20 drops of the root tincture once a day for 4-6 weeks.

★ **Moxibustion** (controlled burning of moxa, an *Artemisia*) over areas of the worst soreness helps warm and soothe all the muscles.

*Step 4. Sedate/Stimulate . . .*

★ A 25-30 drop dose of **St. Joan's wort** tincture stops and prevents muscle aches. Use it before exercise, too.

★ **Massage**, especially from an experienced therapist, releases muscle and joint aches and stimulates the circulation of fresh blood and energy.

*Step 5b.* (See page 169.)

*Step 6. Break and enter . . .*

• Beware invasive diagnostic tests. Many women report enduring endless rounds of scientific tests hoping to find the causes of their menopausal distresses — including aching muscles, crawling skin, dry eyes, burning mouth — with no success and at the price of physical, mental, and emotional distress.

# Birth Control for Menopausal Women

### Step 1. Collect information . . .

Remember your high school chums who unexpectedly had a little baby brother or sister? The biological imperative to reproduce doesn't just die without a struggle. Birth control, never simple or easy, is complicated incredibly by the erratic menses of the menopausal years.

### Step 2. Engage the energy . . .

★ **Barrier methods** are a fairly good choice for the woman in her early menopausal years, though diaphragms may provoke bladder infections; and spermicides (recommended for use with diaphragms, cervical caps, and condoms) may provoke vaginal yeast and itchy vaginal lips.

### Step 3. Nourish and tonify . . .

• During your menopausal years creative sexuality that omits ejaculation in the vagina is a surer form of birth control than it was during your childbearing years. It's also a wonderful way to nourish intimacy in a relationship. And, if your sexual partners are male and in their fifties or older, they may be especially appreciative of sex that doesn't focus on penetration.

★ **Self-pleasuring** is the safest sex for menopausal women: guaranteed not to result in pregnancy! Books and videos can help. (See Betty Dodson's superb offerings, page 41.)

### Step 4. Stimulate/Sedate . . .

★ Other effective, safe means of birth control for the menopausal woman include a mate with a vasectomy, lesbianism, and celibacy.

★ Try an erotic massage encounter instead of intercourse. Use coconut oil as the lubricant. Light candles; buy a bouquet of flowers. Take your time.

### Step 5b. Use drugs . . .

• The Pill (and other hormone-dependent birth control) is not regarded as safe for women over forty.

### Step 6. Break and enter . . .

• If you have an IUD and it causes heavy menstrual periods or flooding, this is a good time to have it removed; flooding, which can increase during the menopausal years, can be a serious threat to your health.

• Sterilization and hysterectomy are offered as a means of birth control when a menopausal woman desires no further children. In some studies, more than half the women reported loss of sex drive and/or decrease in orgasmic responsiveness after tubal ligation or hysterectomy.

# Sex

*"The cycles of fertility pull on you less, my daughter," winks Grandmother Growth. "The urgent cries of your eggs for fertilization are already becoming softer and harder to hear. Do you notice a difference in your desire? You are becoming more than, other than, the woman you were, the woman who was moved to passionate sex when the moon was full and her egg was ripe. You may think your sexual desire is waning, may fear it is leaving you. But observe patiently, my sweet," chuckles Grandmother Growth. "If you will but hold your wise blood inside and stir it in your own cauldron, you will nourish your kundalini, your serpent power, and find yourself, at sixty, passionately sexual with all of life!*

*"But that is for later; for now, let your focus come in. Bring your focus ever inward, in toward your own wholeness. Do not worry if your desire is not attracted outward, is not sparked by others. This will return in time, transformed to fit your transformed self at the end of your menopausal journey.*

*"Right now you have a special opportunity to make peace with your children," admonishes Grandmother Growth. "Make peace with the children you have never given birth to. Make place with the children you have conceived and lost. Make peace with the children you have born and let go of. And then make peace with your own wise child.*

*Grandmother Growth looks into your eyes and you feel the sparks. "You begin your menopausal years by conceiving your own wise child, your baby Crone. Feel your womb making space to cradle you as baby Crone, reserving itself to nourish you as growing Crone, gathering strength to birth you to your crowning as Crone. And know that at your emergence as Crone you will hold inside Child self and Mother self. You will be whole. And you will be sexual."*

As menopause progresses, and ovulation slows and ceases, the last years of "make-a-baby" lust come to an end and you may feel a distinct lessening of libido, or urge to merge with others. This can be especially scary if the image in your mirror no longer seems youthful, or if you look around and don't see any attractive, available partners.

Take heart. Crowned Crones tell us that old women are very, very sexy, but only when they want to be, not when someone else wants them to be. As with many of our menopausal changes, we are offered few role models. We see no lusty crones and so we despair of ever being one. Don't despair. Expand your horizons. (See page 41.)

⚛️

# References & Resources
## Chapter 1: Is This Menopause?

"Alternative Health Care for Women," Patsy Westcott & Leyardia Black, Thorsons, 1987

"Current Obstetric & Gynecologic Diagnosis & Treatment," Appleton/Lang, 1987

"How to Stay Out of the Gynecologist's Office," Fed. of Feminist Women's Health Centers, Women to Women, 1981

"Hysterectomy: Before & After – A Guide to Preventing, Preparing for, and Maximizing Health After," Winnifred Cutler, Harper & Row, 1988

Menstrual Health Foundation, 1-800-845-FLOW

"My Body – My Decision!" Mary Beard, Lindsay & Glade Curtis, HPBooks, 1986

"No More Hysterectomies," Vicki Hufnagel, NAL, 1988

"Our Bodies, Our Selves," Boston Women's Health Book Collective, Simon & Schuster, 1979 (2nd ed.)

"Womancare," Lynda Madaras & Jane Patterson, Avon, 1981

## Sex

"Cultivating Female Sexual Energy," Mantak & Maneewan Chia, Healing Tao, 1986

"Deep Down: New Sensual Writing by Women," Laura Chester, ed., Faber & Faber, 1989

Eve's Garden • Catalog $3 • 119 W. 57th St, Suite 14206, NY, NY 10019

"Female Ejaculation: How-to Video," with Fanny Fatale • $34.95 • Fatale Videos, 526 Castro St., San Francisco, CA 94114

"Ladies Own Erotica," Kensington Ladies' Erotica Society, Ten Speed Press, 1984

"Riding Desire: An Anthology of Erotic Writing," Tee Corinne, ed., Banned Books, 1991

"Sex for One: The Joy of Self Loving," Betty Dodson, Crown, 1992

Sex Over Forty Newsletter, POBox 1600, Chapel Hill, NC 27515

Sexuality Library for Women, catalog $2, from Open Enterprises, 1210 Valencia, San Francisco, CA 94110

"Self-loving Video Portrait," with Betty Dodson • $40 + $5 • Box 1933, Murray Hill Station, NY, NY 10156

Tantra: The Magazine, POBox 79, Torreon, NM 87061 • $4.50 sample

# Mail-Order Books (and Tapes) On Menopause
*all prices include postage*

"A Book About Menopause," Montreal Health Press, CP 1000, Station Place du Parc, Montreal, Quebec, Canada H2W 2N1 • $4 • Excellent!

"Depression is A Feminist Issue," Mature Women's Network, 411 Dunsmuir St, Vancouver, BC, Canada V6B 1X4 • $13.50

"The Gift of Menopause," Anon., 1981, RAJ Publications, POBox 18599, Denver, CO, 80218 • This one is so funny you take it seriously.

"Hearts, Bones, Hot Flashes & Hormones" • $1 • Also, "Taking Hormones and Women's Health: Choices, Risks and Benefits" • $5 • from National Women's Health Network, 1325 G Street NW, Washington, DC 20005

"Herbs for Menopause," Rosemary Gladstar Slick, POBox 420, East Barre, VT 05649 • $6 • Herbal formulas for the menopausal years.

"Menopause, A SelfCare Manual," Santa Fe Health Education Project, POBox 577, Santa Fe, NM 87504-0577 • $7 • **Highly recommended.**

"Menopause" cassette set/3 hours, Women to Women, One Pleasant St, Yarmouth, ME 04096 • $22.95 • Enjoyable.

"Menopause, Me and You," Ann Voda, 1983 • $5 • University of Utah Nursing College, 25 S. Medical Dr., Salt Lake City, UT 84112

"A Positive Look at Menopause," Teacher Training, Planned Parenthood, 800 N Providence, Suite 11, Columbia, MO 65201 • Superb.

"Wise-Woman Archetype: Menopause as Initiation," audio tape, Jean Shinoda Bolen; Sounds True, 735 Walnut St, Boulder, CO 80302 • $12

"Wise Woman Ways for the Menopausal Years" • $13 • Ash Tree Publishing, POBox 64, Woodstock, NY 12498

## Newsletters on Menopause

"Hot Flash," Newsletter of the National Action Forum for Midlife & Older Women, Box 816, Stony Brook, NY, 11790-0609 • $25 yearly

"A Friend Indeed, For Women in the Prime of Life," Newsletter from Box 1710, Champlain, NY, 12919 or Box 515, Place du Parc Station, Montreal, Quebec, Canada H2W 2P1 • $30 for 10 issues. They also offer an annotated bibliography of recommended readings on menopause for $2 plus a stamped, self-addressed envelope.

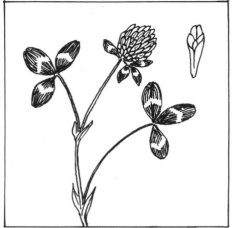

Red Clover — *Trifolium pratense*

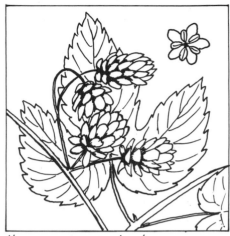

Hops — *Humulus lupulus*

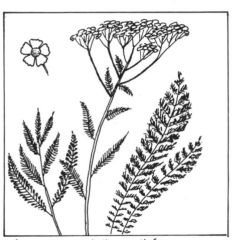

Yarrow — *Achillea millefolium*

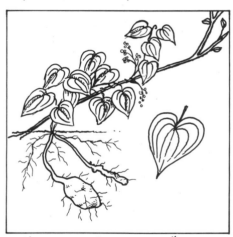

Wild yam — *Dioscorea villosa*

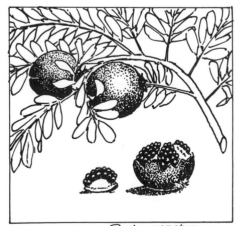

Pomegranate — *Punica granatum*

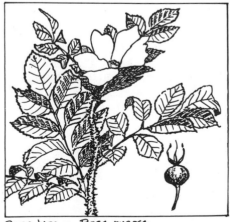

Rose hips — *Rosa rugosa*

# Herbal Allies for
# Women Beginning Menopause

As we know, modern medicine sees menopause as the result of estrogen deficiency. Herbalists who don't question this assumption recommend herbs high in estrogen to menopausal women.

The problem with using estrogen-rich herbs is twofold. First, the hormonal changes of menopause are not restricted to decreasing estrogen levels. Leutinizing hormone (LH) and follicle stimulating hormone (FSH) increase dramatically and stay increased; progesterone decreases and finally disappears; estrogen no longer surges — it declines to a baseline level, then stabilizes. Nor are these changes restricted to the ovaries. Hormonal **Change** takes place during the menopausal years in the liver, the fat cells, the adrenals, the pancreas, the thyroid, and the hypothalamus, too.

Second, while plants do contain plant hormones, no plants have human hormones, so there aren't really any "estrogen-rich" plants. (However, some plants do encourage estrogen production, and some do contain flavonoids, which are estrogen-like.)

Plants hormones are called phytosterols. Phytosterols can be converted to human hormones in the laboratory (birth control pills are based on phytosterols extracted from wild yam roots) or in your body.

Using plants rich in phytosterols is remarkably different from taking hormones, even natural ones such as those used by menopausal women. Phytosterols provide hormonal building blocks, rather than hormones themselves, thus allowing you to create the precise amounts (and combinations) of hormones needed on your unique menopausal journey.

When beginning a regime of ERT (or HRT), it is common to spend months adjusting the dosages of estrogen (and progesterone) until the balance is right. And, since the same dose is taken every day, even though our need for hormones varies daily, there is the stress of eliminating excess estrogen. Excess estrogen unarguably promotes (but does not initiate) breast and reproductive cancers.

When using phytosterol-rich herbs, you don't have to eliminate excess hormones or know exactly what dose to take. With a smorgasbord of choices, the body in her wisdom can create the hormones she needs from the building blocks supplied by the plant. Note that the phytosterol building blocks in plants can be used to decrease hormones (they bind to the hormonal receptor sites) as well as increase hormones (by conversion in the liver).

To date, no increase in breast cancer rates has ever been associated with the use of phytosterol-rich herbs (with the possible exception of licorice); there is, however, a strong correlation between consumption of phytosterol-rich foods (such as yams and soybeans) and decrease in breast cancer rates.

Phytosterols are most concentrated in perennial roots (such as dandelion and ginseng), leaf buds (such as briar rose and black currant) and hard berries (such as vitex and saw palmetto). Your body's access to phytosterols is increased when glycosides, saponins, minerals, and flavonoids are also present in the plant. Renowned hormone-balancing herbs (such as Dong Quai/Dang Gui, black cohosh, and sarsaparilla) contain a dozen or more of these constituents, each of which offers slightly different hormonal building blocks.

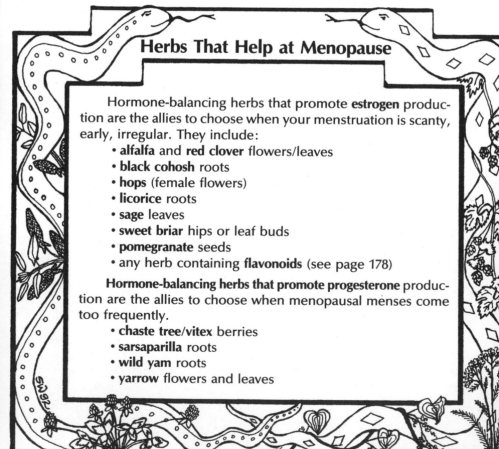

## Herbs That Help at Menopause

Hormone-balancing herbs that promote **estrogen** production are the allies to choose when your menstruation is scanty, early, irregular. They include:
- **alfalfa** and **red clover** flowers/leaves
- **black cohosh** roots
- **hops** (female flowers)
- **licorice** roots
- **sage** leaves
- **sweet briar** hips or leaf buds
- **pomegranate** seeds
- any herb containing **flavonoids** (see page 178)

**Hormone-balancing herbs that promote progesterone** production are the allies to choose when menopausal menses come too frequently.
- **chaste tree/vitex** berries
- **sarsaparilla** roots
- **wild yam** roots
- **yarrow** flowers and leaves

# Phytosterol-Rich Herbs

★ My favorite hormone-balancing herbs for menopausal women are starred.

• Work regularly with **one** — not all, please — of the following herbs for two weeks each month for three or more months, taking the recommended dose 1-3 times a day. Even erratic use of phytosterol-rich plants during the early menopausal years will help nourish your ovaries, adrenals, and pituitary, creating a smoother passage to your Crone's Crowning.

• **Alfalfa,** Luzerne, Luzerne cultivée (*Medicago sativa*) is extraordinarily nourishing but may increase a tendency to hemorrhage. Make a tea of the seeds, or soak as if to sprout and drink the water.

• **Agave** (*Agave americana*) is a desert plant used to balance hormones and, in Chinese medicine, to relieve uterine prolapse. One dose is ¼–1 teaspoon/1-5 ml of fresh juice of the succulent leaves.

★ **Black cohosh,** Schwarze Schlangenwurzel, Cimicifuga (*Cimicifuga racemosa*) is clinically proven to be as effective as ERT in relieving menopausal problems such as hot flashes, sleep disturbances, and irritability. Take the root/rhizome infusion, a swallow at a time, up to a cup/250 ml a day; or use 10-60 drops tincture. (More on page 105.)

• **Black currant,** Schwarze Johannisbeere, Cassis (*Ribes nigrum*) nourishes the adrenals and ovaries and helps prevent urinary tract infections, sore joints, and vascular disorders (including hot flashes). A dose is 10-50 drops of the glycerine macerate of the fresh leaf buds and/or berries.

★ **Black haw,** Amerikanischer Schneeball, Viburnum (*Viburnum prunifolium*) is one of the few hormone-rich herbs highly recommended for women who bleed heavily; it also eases palpitations and menstrual cramps. Sip infusion of the root bark frequently, up to a cup/250 ml a day; or use 15-25 drops of root bark tincture.

★ **Chaste tree** (*Vitex agnus castus*) is considered by some to be *the* herb for menopause. It is an especially important ally for the woman who comes to her menopause early, through natural or induced means. Consistent use of vitex will greatly increase your levels of progesterone and leutinizing hormone (LH). Changes in these two hormones often precede changes in estrogen during the menopausal years. Use a tincture of the fresh or dried berries, 20-40 drops, several times daily. (More, page 107.)

• **Cramp bark** or **Guelder Rose,** Schneeball, Viorne obier (*Viburnum opulis*) is thought of as weak black haw; infusion of the root bark is preferred, 2-3 cups daily/500-750 ml; or 20-40 drops tincture.

★ **Dandelion**, Löwenzahn, Dent-de-lion (*Taraxacum off.*) is rich in plant hormones and a supreme liver nourisher. If you experience one of the most frequent, and least discussed, complaints of menopause — digestive distress — ask dandelion to be your ally. Strengthens bones by improving calcium absorption, too. Dose of the fresh or dried root/leaf tincture is 10-25 drops. Eating the leaves, cooked or raw, and drinking dandelion flower wine is effective, too.

• **Dong Quai/Dang Gui** (*Angelica sinensis*) is one of the most frequently used women's herbs in the world. Use the tincture of fresh or dried roots, 10-40 drops, or infusion of the dried roots, up to a cup/250 ml a day. It supports estrogen production. CAUTION: Dong Quai/Dang Gui increases the possibility of menstrual flooding. (More, page 120.)

• **Devil's club** (*Oplopanax horridum*) is so nourishing to the pancreas that it has been considered a cure for diabetes; laboratory tests confirm its ability to stabilize blood sugar with virtually no side effects. Constipation, sore joints, and menopausal hot flashes also give way to its beneficial influence. Infusion or tincture of the fresh or dried root bark, a cup/250 ml a day, or 5-20 drops, is the dose.

• **False unicorn** (*Chamaelirium luteum*) is a profound ovarian/uterine tonic, especially well-suited to women who flood during their menopausal years. Tincture of the fresh or dried roots is used in 2-5 drop doses several times a day.

★ **Fenugreek**, Bockshornklee, Fenugrec (*Trigonella foenum-graecum*) seeds-are an inexpensive and tasty way to restore your blood sugar balance, nourish your glands, improve your digestion, and incréase your libido. With 27 percent protein and good quantities of EFAs, lecithin, saponins, and phytosterols, fenugreek is an ally treasured by menopausal women. Brew a spoonful of seeds in a cup/250 ml of boiling water for no longer than 15 minutes; drink freely. CAUTION: Fenugreek promotes fertility.

• **Ginseng** (*Panax quinquefolium*) is a heart-healthy herb as well as a hormone balancer. It has an enormous reputation as a reliever of menopausal problems, from flashes to indigestion. Chew on the root or use 5-40 drops of tincture. (More, pages 115-119.)

• **Groundsel**, Gemeines Kreuzkraut, Séneçon Commun (*Senecio vulgaris*) and her sister plant (Jacob's Groundsel), Jakobskraut, Séneçon Jacobée (*Senecio jacobea*) are closely related to liferoot (see below), one of my favorite women's herbs. Prepare the same way as liferoot;

tincture fresh flowers and leaves. (Other parts may be poisonous.) A dose is 10-30 drops, once a day.

★ **Hops**, Hopfen, Houblon grimpant (*Humulus lupulus*) relieves water retention and induces peaceful sleep. It contributes strongly to estrogen production. Make a strong tea of the freshly dried flowers, and sip cold throughout the day, up to a cup a day; better yet, tincture the fresh female flowers and use 5-15 drops once or twice a day.

• **Licorice**, Süssholzwurzel, Réglisse (*Glycyrrhiza glabra*) is a well-known hormonal balancer and anti-inflammatory. CAUTIONS: Licorice may promote certain reproductive cancers. Regular use of licorice can cause high blood pressure and edema (water retention). If you choose to use licorice, drink no more than a cup/250 ml of tea a day. Or chew on a licorice root stick, as needed.

★ **Liferoot** (*Senecio aureus*) promotes menstrual and menopausal ease. Use 5-10 drops of the fresh flower tincture, once a day only. (More, page 109.)

• **Motherwort**, Herzgespan, Agripaume cardiaque (*Leonurus cardiaca*) is a magnificent herbal ally for the menopausal woman, for all women. She moderates hot flashes and night sweats, eases emotional swings, strengthens the heart, and relieves cramping. Use tincture of the flowering tops, taking 5-15 drops several times a day, as needed. (More, pages 113-115.)

★ **Nettle**, Brennessel, Ortie (*Urtica dioica* or *U. urens*) is my dearest ally. She does it all: keeps my bones strong, my heart healthy, and my menopausal journey on a smooth road. There is no better herb for restoring kidney and adrenal functioning. (An occasional post-menopausal woman has found her menses returning with regular use of sister spinster stinging nettle.) I drink nettle infusion freely and eat the greens whenever I can. (More, page 177.)

• **Peony** (*Paeonia albiflora* or *P. officinalis*) has hormone-rich roots, but poisonous flowers and leaves. Use tincture of the fresh or dried roots, 1-25 drops at a time, several times daily, to establish menstrual regularity, ease cramps, and soothe emotional swings. Frequently combined with Dong Quai/Dang Gui.

★ **Pomegranate** (*Punica granatum*) is a fruit rich in fertility associations. The seeds contain estrone, a form of estrogen. One researcher found 1.7 mg estrone in 100 grams (about 3 ounces). How to take them? Just eat them instead of spitting them out when you consume the fruit. Or whir them in a blender with other fruit to make a smoothie. You can also grind them and infuse in oil to make your own estrogen cream.

• **Raspberry**, Himbeere, Framboisier (*Rubus species*) is an important hormonal ally during the childbearing and the menopausal years. Drink the leaf infusion hot or cold, or take 20-35 drops of a glycerin macerate twice a day. (See **Rose**, below.)

★ **Red clover**, Rotklee, trèfle des prés (*Trifolium praetense*), like alfalfa, is highly nourishing, cancer curative, and a calming reliever of menopausal distresses such as sore joints, anxiety, and energy loss. Red clover may contribute to blood thinning (a helpful thing if you want to prevent strokes, but a liability if you are flooding). Use infusions of dried blossoms freely, or make a vinegar with fresh flowers.

★ The **Rose family** contains many members eager to help menopausal women: raspberry, strawberry, sweet briar, and hawthorn. Any part of any rose can be used to ease headaches, relieve dizziness, nourish the nerves and heart, invigorate the entire being, remedy menstrual cramps, strengthen the bones, and moderate mood and hormonal swings during the **Change**. Rose hips are an excellent source of flavonoids.

★ **Sage**, Salbei, Sauge officinale (*Salvia officinalis*), also called garden sage, relieves night sweats, depression, trembling, and dizziness. It clearly promotes estrogen production, and may lower FSH and LH surges during the menopausal years. Infuse the leaves, dilute, and sip throughout the day. Or tincture fresh leaves and take 5-15 drops as needed. (More, pages 111-112.)

• **Sarsaparilla**, Sarsaparillawurzel, Salsepareille (*Smilax officinalis or S. regelii* or other species) is an old favorite of menopausal women. Confusion reigns when you attempt to purchase sarsaparilla (pronounced sas-prilla) as there are numerous species, some of which are much more effective than others. Jamaican is considered the best, with Mexican and Honduran following closely. Use infusion of dried root, ½–1 cup/125-250 ml; or 10-30 drops of fresh or dried root tincture. Sarsaparilla noticeably supports progesterone production.

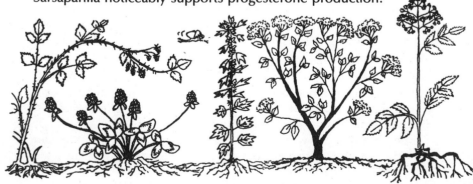

• **Saw palmetto** (*Serenoa serrulata*) is best known as an herb for correcting enlarged prostate (BPH) but it is worth consideration by menopausal women for its reputed ability to prevent atrophy of ovarian, vaginal, breast, and bladder tissue. It has a long-standing reputation as an aphrodisiac. Use infusion of dried berries, ½–1 cup/125-250 ml; or, better yet, if you live along the Gulf Coast, tincture the fresh berries, and take 10-25 drops two or three times a day.

★ **Sweet briar** or dog-rose, Hagrose, Eglantier (*Rosa canina* or *R. pendulina*) is a powerful menopausal ally rarely mentioned in modern herbals. Use leaf bud glycerin macerate, or a tea of the fruits/hips. Take in any quantity. (See also **Rose**.)

• **Wild yam** (*Dioscorea villosa* and all 500 related species) is exceptionally useful for promoting the production of progesterone. Wild yam root strengthens the liver, soothes the nerves, and eases menstrual pain. Progesterone cream derived from wild yam has been shown to reverse osteoporosis. Use dried root infusion, ½–1 cup/125-250 ml daily; or dried root tincture, 10-30 drops.

• **Yarrow**, Schafgarbe, Millefeuille (*Achillea millefolium*) is thought to be especially active in creating progesterone. Yarrow also remedies bladder infections, incontinence, and flooding, but may increase sweating with hot flashes. One herbalist offers the observation that yarrow is excellent for tough, independent women who don't talk about their problems. Sip tea or infusion of the dried flowers as desired. To improve flavor, add some fennel seeds. Or try a tincture of the fresh flowering tops, 5-10 drops, two or three times a day. Try the flower essence when you feel drained.

How to ingest your ally? If hot drinks trigger your hot flashes, take your teas and infusions at room temperature or chilled. Alcohol-sensitive women will want to tincture their herbs in vinegar rather than vodka; a teaspoon/5 ml of vinegar tincture is about equal to 10-20 drops alcohol tincture. Always put your dose of tincture (vodka or vinegar) in half a glass of water before you take it.

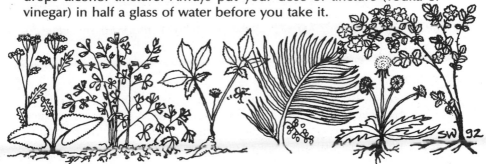

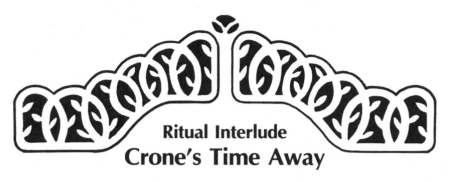

### Ritual Interlude
# Crone's Time Away

The first stage of self-initiation as Crone is isolation. Just as the menstruating woman chooses isolation or has isolation thrust upon her in the form of painful periods, the menopausal woman may choose isolation or may "become" the victim as her husband leaves her, her children grow up, and her erratic moods alienate her former friends. Chosen or not, manifested subtly as depression or dramatically as hysteria, isolation stalks the menopausal woman and carries her into her Crone's Time Away.

As menopausal changes increase, our physical processes lead us into isolation. We want to sleep alone so the constant wakings and cover tossings can be guilt-free. We want to be alone so we can undress and dress as flushes and flashes and sweats of heated energy flow through our bodies. We want to be alone to face our **Change**, to embrace the chaos and our own darkness.

In isolation we hear, perhaps for the first time, the voice of our own needs, our own desires. In isolation we have the time, perhaps never before available, to tend to our own needs and our own wants.

Your Crone's Time Away begins with a ritual of isolation. This may be done by yourself or with others. The following is one possibility. It is designed to be done with your family and close friends as a way of telling them that your need for privacy and isolation is not a rejection of them but a claiming of yourself. It may open into an actual time of isolation, a vacation, a separate room or cabin, or it may create an aura of awe around you that will allow you to feel into your moods and needs without the constant pressure to tend to others.

\*     \*     \*     \*     \*

Gather with your family and friends in a public place, the noisier the better, symbolizing the busyness of your life. Walk from this place to a quieter, more isolated area, outside or in, symbolizing the quiet space you are creating for your transformation.

Facing each other, join hands, and hum. Don't worry about how you sound. Pay attention to your breath and your feet and let the hum vibrate through you.

Invite the energies of the seven directions to be present with you: east, south, west, north, below, above, and within. Face the east and ask each person to say one word that evokes the east (such as dawn, flight, laughter, inspiration). Do the same for the south (summer, cauldron, protection) and the west (death, ocean, emotion) and the north (unknown, crystal, vision, earth). You may wish to say: "Energy of the east (south, west, north) be here now."

Ask everyone to bend their knees and put their hands on the earth and breathe out with a sigh. Ask everyone to stretch, fingertips to the sky, and inhale fully. Facing each other again, put both hands on your heart, close your eyes and honor the space of within, the vibral core.

Using your own words, speak to each person. Stand in front of this person while you speak. "You are my lover (daughter, friend, son, sister, mate). I take great joy in pleasing you. I feel great power in making your life easy and abundant. In the next years I will be busy finding my way to myself as crone. This way takes me through menopause, the great **Change**. What I will find I know not now. And how I will change I know not now. Of this I am sure, however, my love and affection for you will not change. Together we affirm this bond.

"Yet I must take this journey of all journeys alone. I ask now for your blessing on me as I begin my journey. I ask you to acknowledge that I need to have my Crone's Time Away. I am growing. Let me go now so this growth does not wrench me from your grasp."

Speak in your own way, in song or dance, in poetry or a prepared script, to each person or everyone; they need not respond.

When you are complete, join hands again and begin to hum. Let the hum go on as long as it feels right. Lift your arms to the sky and breathe out. Place your palms on the earth and breathe in. Turn to the north and send a feeling of gratefulness for the qualities of the north that you carry with you (you may each speak them aloud). Turn to the west, south, and east with gratitude and awareness of their attributes you already carry. You may wish to say: "Thank you, energies of the north (west, south, east); hail and farewell."

Drop hands. Leave the circle by yourself. Spend the night alone. In the silence you may hear Grandmother Growth whispering in your ear.

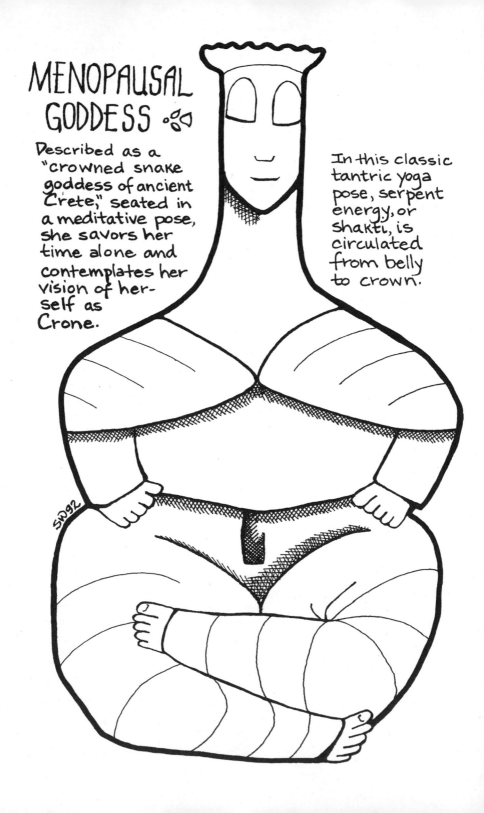

# MENOPAUSAL GOODESS

Described as a "crowned snake goddess of ancient Crete," seated in a meditative pose, she savors her time alone and contemplates her vision of herself as Crone.

In this classic tantric yoga pose, serpent energy, or shakti, is circulated from belly to crown.

SDW92

# This Is Menopause!
## Journey Into Change

*"Pay attention, now," Grandmother Growth says, taking your hand and holding your gaze. "The Change known as menopause deserves your full attention.*

*"Pay attention now, and relax. Focus, allow, observe, surrender. Your egg basket empties; your memory basket grows heavier.*

*"Memories are sweeping through you, great granddaughter, like lightning flashes, leaving you shaken and trembling, sweating and panting. Memories too gossamer to catch with words are weaving themselves into your nights and shattering the patterns of your days. Fragments of melodies, half-seen gestures, sketches, muted drifts of color emerge from your memory. All the wild passions of the Maiden are restored to you. All those Maiden things you left behind or pushed aside when you became Mother-woman, return to you now, enriched.*

*"Do these memories crowd painfully into your head? Do they send your heart racing? Do they make you weep? Sweep you off your feet? Leave you wondering what it would feel like to jump off a high bridge? Take my hand, dear one. Let us walk and talk."*

There is no doubt left in your mind. Your menstrual cycles are coming to an end. You are in the midst of your menopausal climax years.

During the year or so before the very last period (and the year or so afterward) many women experience some type of menopausal **Change**, such as hot flashes, dizziness, heart palpitations, emotional uproar, sleep disturbances, and/or headaches.

Since many of us celebrate our mid-life feeling more happily in control of our lives than ever before, giving in to menopausal **Change** isn't easy. The desire to use anything, drugs or herbs or whatever, to avoid disruption of our normal life pattern is strong; it comes from within and is reinforced by society. Why resist?

Wise Woman ways, the women's mystery stories, and a host of helpful herbal allies offer us a greater vision. They let us share in a story where hot flashes and wild heart beats are honored as metamorphic processes in a woman's greatest transformation, her crowning as Crone, with remedies to aid this process rather than attempt to stop it.

Wise Woman stories say that menopause is an initiation and that initiation begins with a period of isolation. The grandmothers tell me that, as a menopausal woman, I need to draw inward, move away from outside responsibility, and isolate myself. Menopausal hot flashes, fatigue, headaches, and emotional outbursts become allies of wholeness instead of problems if I allow them to lead me to seek time alone where I can focus inward on my **Change**.

Without knowledge of the women's mystery stories, without the reassurance of herbal allies, a woman may feel alone and unsupported in her disturbing and "pointless" changes. (In a recent issue of a national magazine, two mid-life women made fun of their flashing friend for not taking ERT and "avoiding all that fuss and bother.") She sees no reason to endure **Change**.

She is told (erroneously) that her **Change** is responsible for a list of horrors, from death by heart attack to crumbling bones, from wrinkles and grey hair to loss of sex appeal and libido. There is no Grandmother Growth to guide her through this immense, frightening metamorphosis, to show her the green gifts of nature that strengthen her heart and bones, soften her skin and sex.

Science defines the problem (menopause results from lack of estrogen) and prescribes the remedy (take estrogen replacement) and reassures us that we don't have to mature, to become wise women. We can remain bound to our (and society's) idea of who we ought to be, instead of exploring who we really are.

If I took ERT would I be able to make room for transformation? take time for solitude? give myself uninterrupted stretches of focused self-loving? encounter, nourish, and sanctify myself as a wise and silly grandmother, a wrinkled wild woman, a lawless fierce crone? My menopausal metamorphosis deserves as much attention as I can give it. And I am not that rare woman who gives herself these gifts without the daily urgings of her body and feelings.

So I don't take ERT. I choose to let the "problems" of my menopause give me the opportunity to claim all parts of myself, even those that are awkward, ugly, old, out of control, and afraid of death. By passing consciously through menopause, by embracing this **Change** in my life, by nourishing myself with green allies, I can complete myself as woman — reclaiming myself as maiden, redefining myself as mother, *and* knowing myself as crone — so the grandmothers tell me.

*"Take my hand, dear one. I will soothe your head, calm your heart, stabilize your grounding, and then teach you to fly. Take my hand, now. You are in the midst of Change."*

# Flashes and Flushes and Chills

*"Give me your full attention, young Crone," says Grandmother Growth in a voice deep and resonant. "For you will pay attention, I assure you, when your menopausal Change lets loose lightning-like hot flashes and waves of energy that free your feelings and stir your spirit. As you hold the wise blood inside more and more, menstruating less and less, strong energies will move in you. The women's mystery teachings of menopause urge you to take time off to adapt to these energies, to take, symbolically or actually, real Crone's Time Away and allow those hot flashes and sleepless nights to guide you into metamorphosis and initiation."*

Hot flashes! The archetypal distress of menopause. After years of being told to hide my menstrual blood (my womanness), after years of successfully being in public without anyone suspecting that I was a menstruating woman, suddenly I am revealed.

The blood that no longer comes so regularly flowing from my womb now rushes to my face, flushing my skin and covering me in a damp shimmer. I feel at the mercy of the flash, which takes me when it decides, and gives no warning (I am reminded of my labor pains, of sexual arousal/release).

My hot flash tells the world, I am sure, that I am woman (vulnerable and invisible). Not just woman, but old woman (much more vulnerable, much more invisible). I live in a civilized country where I am expected to go through a powerful **Change** as though it were nothing, and where my survival may depend on how I look. I am urged by both outer and inner voices to to do whatever I can to appear young: dye my hair, have a face lift, take calcium supplements, and use estrogen to eliminate the obvious sign of my **Change** — hot flashes.

If I lived in a world safe for women, in a matrifocal culture guided by the wisdom of the crones, I would cherish my hot flashes and cherish myself as I experienced them. I would be taught to respect my flashes as part of the gestation of myself in the fiery womb of menopause/metamorphosis. I would be seen as baby Crone. I would learn how to thrill to the waves of energy (prana, kundalini, chi, life force) as they rush through me, flashing, flushing, pulsing. I would have guides and role models and stories and herbal and animal allies to help me. I would be urged/allowed to take my Crone's Year Away. I would *want* to be a wise old woman. I wouldn't want to be cured of my hot flashes or delay my old age.

I wonder, did the matrifocal nations, the ancient wise women, have remedies to relieve hot flashes? Even if they respected and valued the transformative power of their flashes and flushes, I'm sure they would have had wonderful remedies to help the woman distressed by her flashes, for the Wise Woman way seeks both/and solutions. I think they used some of the same herbs and home remedies I do, and you can, too.

# Hot Flashes

*Step 0. Do Nothing . . .*

★ My baby Crone friend Marie Summerwood gives herself a **"Crone's Moment Away."** When she flashes, she closes her eyes and focuses in, taking a moment ("It can seem like a year . . .") away.

*Step 1. Collect information . . .*

Hot flashes are virtually synonymous with menopause. The vast majority of women will have had at least one hot flash by the age of sixty.

Hot flashes are regarded as a symptom of estrogen deficiency by the modern medical profession, and are treated with estrogen replacement. But women with severe hot flashes have been found to have about the same amount of estrogen in their blood as women who have mild (or nonexistent) flashes. In fact, one small study found that, while the intensity of the hot flashes was abated in women who took supplemental estrogen, the overall duration of their hot flashes was more than twice as long as the average (five years rather than two).

The far greater hormonal change, and the change more likely responsible for hot flashes, is the elevation of the hormones FSH and LH during (and after) the menopausal years. These pituitary hormones can be 1300 percent greater during the menopausal years than before.

*The frequency, intensity, and duration of hot flashes is unique to each woman in her menopausal years.*

During a hot flash, flushes of heat sweep the upper body (and often the face), reddening the skin and prompting free perspiration. The reddening may be blotchy or even; the perspiration slight or copious.

A single hot flash usually lasts from a few seconds to four minutes, occasionally for fifteen minutes, rarely more than an hour.

*"At 56, I've only missed two periods. I've had two rounds of very intense hot flashes — each round lasting six weeks — a year apart."*

Hot flashes may occur at irregular intervals, every 60-90 minutes (the adrenal cycle), or only at certain times of the day and night. (Sadja Greenwood, author of *Menopause Naturally*, says flashes are most common between 6 and 9 PM.) Women have experienced up to 30 hot flashes a day, but the average is less than one a day.

After a hot flash that provokes enough perspiration to dampen (or soak) your clothes, you may experience a profound chill.

Estimates of women who have hot flashes during the menopausal years range from 50 percent to 85 percent. Some men have hot flashes during their late forties and early fifties. And an occasional woman experiences cold flashes.

Of the women who do have hot flashes during the menopausal years, 80 percent have them for between two months and two years. A small percentage have flashes into their seventies and eighties. And about 20 percent experience flashes for a full decade after the last menstrual flow.

When menopause is induced (by surgical removal of the ovaries, chemotherapy, or radiation), nearly 100 percent of the women experience hot flashes. In women who refuse post-operative hormonal drugs (ERT/HRT), the period of hot flashes is, as with biological menopause, almost always under two years, though the flashes are more frequent and more intense than those of women achieving menopause naturally. (In the process of writing this book, I met quite a few women who refused post-operative ERT. All were happy with their decision and were in good health.)

Thinner women experience more rapid changes in their estrogen and FSH/LH levels during the menopausal years, and, therefore, are more likely to experience strong hot flashes. Fat cells moderate the hormonal levels and slowing the rapid rise of FSH/LH.

From an energy viewpoint, a hot flash is a release of kundalini (cosmic) electricity, which "rewires" the nervous system, making it capable of transferring and moving powerful healing energies for the entire community. (Community healing and peace-keeping are two important tasks of the Crone. Long-term use of ERT may prevent the emergence of these energies.)

*"Sometimes there's a blip, then a flush whooooooshes up to my head; other times it comes on with no warning — flash! — and I'm covered in dampness. Some hover around my neck; some cover my whole torso. But all of them are HOT."*

### Step 2. Engage the energy . . .

• **Keep cool.** Drink plenty of water and herbal infusions. Turn the thermostat down. Eat smaller meals, more frequently. Walk away from aggravating situations. Soak your feet. Think cool. Let your grey hairs blow cool thoughts along your spine. Wear silk. Envision a waterfall. Put ice on your cheeks.

★ Judyth Reichenberg-Ullman, a naturopathic physician, finds **homeopathic remedies** effective 80 percent of the time in relieving menopausal symptoms. One of her favorite remedies for women with hot flashes is *Lachesis.* Try *Lachesis* when the flashes/flushes emanate from the top of your head, are worse just before sleep and immediately upon awakening, and are accompanied by sweating, headaches, or easily irritated skin.

• Other useful **homeopathic remedies** include:
  ☞ *Sepia*: your flashes make you feel weak, nauseated, exhausted, and depressed.
  ☞ *Pulsatilla*: you flash less outdoors, but your flashes are often followed by intense chills and emotional uproar.
  ☞ *Valeriana*: your face flushes strongly during the flash, and you have intense sweating and sleeplessness.
  ☞ *Ferrum metallicum*: your flashes are sudden; your general health is good but ordinary activities bring exhaustion.
  ☞ *Sulfuricum acidicum*: your flashes include profuse sweating and trembling, are worse in evenings or with exercise.
  ☞ *Sanguinaria*: your cheeks are red and burning, feet and hands hot.
  ☞ *Belladonna*: the flash centers on your face, which burns and turns bright red; you are restless, agitated, and have palpitations.

• Put several drops of essential oil of **calamus/sweet flag** in a hot bath and soak. . . . Or put some on a handkerchief and inhale as you begin to flash.

• Essential oils of **basil** or **thyme** also ease flashes when inhaled or used in a bath or foot rub or mixed with massage oil.

• **Biofeedback** helps you learn how to consciously dilate and constrict your blood vessels. (Especially recommended for women who also have menopausal migraines.)

*"I started having irregular flashes when I was 44. Usually they would come when I was just starting to bleed, which I thought quite unfair. One or the other, isn't that the way it's supposed to be?"*

• Hot flashes have been compared by many women to three major experiences: anger, orgasm, and enlightenment. All are accompanied by the release in the nervous system of powerful kundalini energies. The **Kundalini Meditation** helps you contact these sensations and feelings and their connections to your flashes. It is best done after you have already had several hot flashes. (See page 60.)

### Step 3. Nourish and tonify . . .

• Hot flashes deplete vitamin B, vitamin C, magnesium, and potassium. Frequent use of **red clover** or **oatstraw** infusions will replace these needed nutrients.

• **Exercise** directly decreases hot flashes by decreasing the amount of circulating LH and FSH, by nourishing and tonifying the hypothalamus, and by raising endorphin levels (which plummet with hot flashing). As little as 20 minutes three times a week can reduce flashes significantly.

*"It is now four years since menstruation stopped; the flashes are getting lighter, coming less often."*

• **Herbal remedies** for women with hot flashes include plants that **cool the system**, such as chickweed, elder, and violet; plants that **nourish the liver**, such as dandelion and yellow dock; and plants rich in **phytosterols**, such as black cohosh. Choose one from each group and make your own special blend for your menopausal journey (see boxes pages 63, 64, 65).

### Step 4. Sedate/Stimulate . . .

• Indulge yourself with a beautiful hand **fan** (if it's old, fantasize about the last menopausal woman who cooled herself with it) or try a pocket/purse-sized battery-run breeze-maker.

• **Cologne**, which is mostly alcohol, and therefore highly evaporative, can help you get cool, cool, cool. Pour some on a hankie; enclose tightly in a plastic bag; off you go. When the flash strikes, you're ready to mop it up, revive yourself, and smell great.

• **Baths** are so relaxing. Use menopause as an excuse to jump in. If you are flashing hourly, try a bath with 3 ounces/80 ml of rubbing alcohol in it. Ah. . . . And there's also the "at-home ocean cure": Pour 1 cup/250 ml sea salt in a hot bath. Lounge and envision an island paradise.

*"And at the height of it I was having five hot flashes during the night and one every hour during the day."*

# Kundalini Meditation

*Sit or lie down in a private, safe space.*

Bring all your attention to your breath. As you breathe out, imagine waves flowing out of you with your breath. Breathe out waves of water, of energy, of color, of sound. Allow these waves to flow out of you. Notice where you are tensing, pushing, trying to make the waves happen. And let go, let the waves flow out easily with your breath. Feel the gentle pulsations of the waves deep inside yourself. Feel every cell of your being pulsing peacefully and joyfully with these waves.

When you are ready, begin to draw red vibrations in with your inhalation. Envision yourself filling up with glowing, sparkling, swirling, hot, steaming red. Feel fast spirals of red boiling inside; feel slow vortices of red churning inside. Then breathe out and feel the red flowing out of you in waves. Dissolve into the waves as you breathe out.

With each inhalation, increase the intensity, sharpen the sensation of red: let it be hotter, richer, deeper, more vivid, more consuming. Inhale sun-ripened tomato flesh, sweet cherry juice dribbling down your chin, a sudden gush of menstrual blood blossoming on your clothes. Inhale the seething red sun as it sets into a heaving red sea. Inhale the essence of red roses. Inhale the color of strawberries, the scent of raspberries, the sensation of red satin. Inhale red.

Then breathe it all out. Pause. Feel the emptiness.

Inhale red. Say, out loud or silently: "Sometimes I get upset inside." Blow out any remaining air as though you were blowing out a candle. Pause in the emptiness. Breathe in red and say it again: "Sometimes I get upset inside." Blow. Pause. Inhale. "Sometimes I get upset inside."

Blow, pause, inhale, and say, in big red letters: "Sometimes I get angry." Blow. Pause. Inhale. "Sometimes I get angry." Blow. Pause. Inhale. "Sometimes I get angry."

Exhale forcibly. Pause in the emptiness. Inhale red. Say, with passion: "Sometimes I feel furious." Again: blow, pause, inhale, and say: "Sometimes I feel furious." Out, quiet, in, with intensity, say: "Sometimes I feel furious."

Exhale strongly, pause, inhale bright red, yell: "Sometimes I am enraged." (Three times.)

Blow hard, rest, inhale fully, and say: "Sometimes I want to scream, and kick and beat my fists." (Three times.)

Exhale, wait, inhale red. As you inhale, say, out loud or silently: "Sometimes I have very sexual thoughts." Breathe out, pause in the emptiness; breathe in red and say it again: "Sometimes I have very sexual thoughts." Exhale, pause, inhale, and say it again: "Sometimes I have very sexual thoughts."

Blow, rest, inhale velvet red, and acknowledge: "Sometimes I only want to think about my pleasure." Breathe out and pause. Inhale satin red and say: "Sometimes I only want to think about my pleasure." Empty your lungs and wait a moment before you inhale lipstick red and say, once more: "Sometimes I only want to think about my pleasure."

Breathe out. Rest. As you inhale blood red say: "Sometimes my entire being is nothing but waves of sensation." Blow, pause, breathe in tropical sunset red and say, "Sometimes my entire being is nothing but unbounded waves of sensation." Empty, wait, inhale the fresh red petals of a rose and say: "Sometimes my entire being is nothing but waves of sensation."

Exhale, sighing deeply. Pause.

Breathe slowly in and out for three breaths. Let the air you breathe be crystalline: clear, sharp, compelling. Let your third inhalation be deeply nourishing, your third exhalation completely freeing. Pay special attention to the energy in your root chakra (lower pelvis or sitting area).

When you are ready, open your eyes. Get up. Stretch. Record your impressions in words or colors.

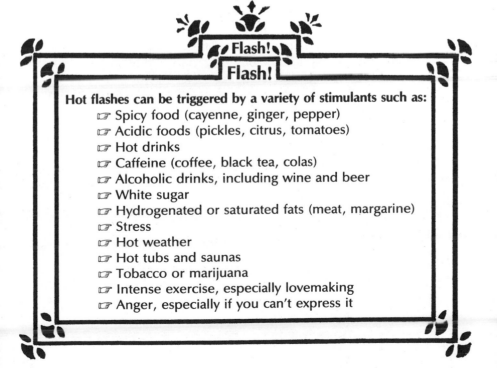

**Flash! Flash!**

Hot flashes can be triggered by a variety of stimulants such as:
- ☞ Spicy food (cayenne, ginger, pepper)
- ☞ Acidic foods (pickles, citrus, tomatoes)
- ☞ Hot drinks
- ☞ Caffeine (coffee, black tea, colas)
- ☞ Alcoholic drinks, including wine and beer
- ☞ White sugar
- ☞ Hydrogenated or saturated fats (meat, margarine)
- ☞ Stress
- ☞ Hot weather
- ☞ Hot tubs and saunas
- ☞ Tobacco or marijuana
- ☞ Intense exercise, especially lovemaking
- ☞ Anger, especially if you can't express it

• **What to wear** takes on a whole new significance when you are faced with the possibility of being both intensely hot and thoroughly chilled several times a day. The crones I talked to gave me these hints:

☞ Dress in layers so you can remove and replace clothing easily.

☞ Try silk or miracle fibers for the layer next to your skin. Cotton and nylon hold the sweat when you flash and can contribute significantly to the chill that follows. (Damp, wet cotton; ugh.) Silk and miracle fibers let the moisture evaporate.

☞ Wear loose clothes; no turtlenecks or belts. It is not uncommon to feel suffocated during a hot flash. How about a skirt?

☞ Sweaters and blouses that button in the front are a must; pullovers leave you feeling disarrayed when you try to get out of them quickly.

• Bee pollen and algae may contain hormonal precursors; some women report good results taking small daily amounts of either during the menopausal years.

*Step 5a. Use supplements . . .*

★ **Vitamin E** supplements have a well-documented and long-standing reputation as a remedy for hot flashes. Vitamin E helps reverse and prevent dry vaginal tissues and heart disease as well. Doses of 200-600 IU (sometimes even 1200 IU) are taken daily for periods ranging from a month to several years to help relieve hot flashes. The most important thing to look for in buying vitamin E supplements is freshness. Taking rancid vitamin E will have the opposite effect of your intent. For easiest digestion, try taking your supplement as part of a meal containing at least a spoonful of vegetable oil; or use the dry form of vitamin E. CAUTIONS: Vitamin E supplements over 100 IU are generally contra-indicated for women with diabetes, high blood pressure, or rheumatic heart conditions; those taking digitalis or anti-coagulants; and anyone experiencing vision disturbances. If you suddenly have a menses or two after taking vitamin E supplements, stop, or reduce dosage.

• Selenium is a synergistic partner of vitamin E; 15-50 mg daily increases effectiveness of vitamin E.

★ B vitamins, especially $B_2$, $B_6$, and $B_{12}$, are needed in very large quantities during the years you are flashing.

• Bioflavonoid supplements, 250 mg 5-6 times daily, help relieve hot flashes. Hesperidin, a type of bioflavonoid and a component of vitamin C, is also recommended for alleviating hot flashes. Dosage is 1000 mg daily.

*"Experiencing menopause at such an early age (41) is embarrassing. I feel inhibited about discussing it with my peers. Even if menopause is normal, I feel abnormal."*

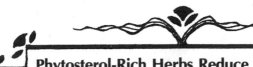

## Phytosterol-Rich Herbs Reduce Frequency and Intensity of Flashes

★ A scientifically controlled study done in 1988 showed **black cohosh** (a phytosterol-rich herb) to be as effective — both objectively, by tests of hormone levels, and subjectively, as reported by the women — as ERT in reducing menopausal problems. Use 30-60 drops of the root tincture several times daily.

◇ Herbalist Silena Heron's basic menopausal formula (which she'd adjust to fit your specific needs) includes ten phytosterol-rich herbs: two parts chaste tree, one part each motherwort, false unicorn, Dong Quai/Dang Gui, garden sage, and St. Joan's wort, and one-half part each black cohosh, licorice, black haw, alfalfa, and dandelion. If you want to try a formula like this and can't get every one of the herbs, just leave some out, remembering that any *one* of these herbs may be plenty.

◇ Rina Nissim, Swiss herbalist and author of *Natural Healing in Gynecology*, suggests this menopausal combination: tincture or glycerine macerate of black currant buds, raspberry leaves, sweet briar (rose) hips and leaf buds. Use one or all, in equal parts, 30-40 drops twice a day.

◇ Gregorita Rodriguez, a *curandera* in New Mexico, recommends these herbs to women troubled by hot flashes: yerba de zorillo/wormseed (*Chenopodium ambrosioides*), escoba de la víbora/yellow snakeweed (*Gutierrezia sarothrae*), and yerba mansa/lizard's tail (*Anemopsis californica*). Use equal parts of the dried leaves or fresh whole plants. Boil quickly, then steep for ten or more minutes. Take up to three cups/750 ml daily.

★ Make phytosterol-rich **fenugreek** seed tea your wake-up and good-night brew; you'll have fewer hot flashes and flushes and, when you do flash, your sweat will smell like sweet maple syrup.

◇ Grandfather herbalist Dr. Christopher uses a variety of phytosterol-rich herbs in "Chagese," his formula for "the change": American ginseng, licorice, sarsaparilla, black cohosh, false unicorn, blessed thistle, and spikenard.

◇ Soy beans and yams contain a preformed steroidal nucleus, as do most whole grains. That means *you* get a nucleus/center around which your body can easily create steroids/hormones when you eat them.

• See pages 45-49 for dosages of phytosterol-rich plants.

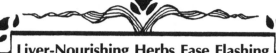

## Liver-Nourishing Herbs Ease Flashing

★ **Dandelion**, Lowenzahn, Dent-de-lion (*Taraxacum officinale*) root is a famous and favorite liver tonic and nourisher wherever it grows, and that's just about everywhere. Regular use of any part of dandelion, from flowers to roots, can offer us easier times with hot flashes by helping the liver metabolize surplus LH and FSH.

Dandelion is especially recommended for the woman who experiences peculiar sensations on her skin during the menopausal years, and for the woman whose digestive system feels the **Change**. A dose is 10-25 drops of the root tincture, or a small spoonful of the root/leaf vinegar, taken 1-3 times a day.

◇ **Ho Shou Wu** (*Polygonum multiflorum*) roots are nearly as storied as ginseng under their popular name: Fo-ti-tieng. An infusion taken frequently not only nourishes the liver but also restores energy, prevents premature aging and adult onset diabetes, benefits the bones, and strengthens the kidneys.

◇ **Yellow dock** (*Rumex crispus*) root tincture or vinegar and the seeds of the **milk thistle** (*Syllibum*) thistle are also liver nourishers of note. *Syllibum* is something of a celebrity for restoring health to poisoned and "helpless" livers; try it for acute distress. Yellow dock is a common weed of roadsides; use 10-20 drops daily for long-term strengthening and health of your liver.

◇ Other liver-nourishing herbs include: all parts of chicory (*Cichorium intybus*), oatstraw, and all parts of burdock. (Coffee, comfrey root, and more than an ounce of alcohol a day distress the liver.)

*"I'm 51 and in the past year I had extreme hot flashes for 7 months. I didn't really do anything about them and they've eased up the past couple of months. They did make life more interesting."*

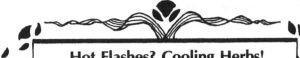

## Hot Flashes? Cooling Herbs!

★ **Chickweed**, Vogelmiere, Stellaire (*Stellaria media*) is often disregarded as a medicinal plant, yet woman after woman has commented to me about the relief she has had during the menopausal years from regular use of chickweed tincture. A dose of 25-40 drops of fresh plant tincture taken once or twice a day helps nourish and stabilize the glandular temperature control system, thus reducing the severity and frequency of hot flashes. Results are generally evident within a week or two of regular use. Regular use of chickweed tincture now can help prevent vaginal dryness later on in your menopausal years.

• **Elder flower**, Holunder, Sureau (*Sambucus* species) tincture is the specific herb for resetting the body's thermostat. When frequent hot flashes or night sweats interrupt your life (and you haven't yet figured out how to take your Crone's Time Away), try using 25-50 drops of fresh elder blossom tincture several times a day. (There is no overdose, so use all you want.) Results should be noticeable within a few days.

• **Violet**, Veilchen, Violette (*Viola* species) leaves not only cool the overheated menopausal woman, but also help protect her reproductive tissues from cancer. Use the dried leaves to make an infusion; drink freely, at least a cup/250 ml a day.

• Other cooling herbal allies for menopausal women include oatstraw, mint, and seaweeds, all parts of all the mallows (*Malva* species), and the flowers and leaves of any hibiscus (*Hibiscus*).

*"I'm 48 now; the year I turned 44 I began to have full body sweats on a daily basis, but only in the spring and fall."*

### Step 5b. Use drugs . . .

• Supplemental estrogen (ERT) is the drug of choice to relieve hot flashes. The woman catapulted into menopause by surgery, radiation, or chemotherapy may be told her hot flashes will be "unbearable" without ERT. While ERT does alleviate hot flashes for many women, practitioners around the country tell me of women taking ERT for years and continuing to have intense flashes. There is actually little benefit in taking ERT solely for relief of hot flashes.

If you do decide to use ERT, conservative recommendations suggest use of the lowest dose you find effective, taken as briefly as possible. Use liver-nourishing herbs, like dandelion, while on ERT or HRT. Interface with phytosterol-rich herbs as you taper off, optimally within thirteen months.

• Other drugs used to control hot flashes include progestins such as Norlutin or Proveramay (side effects include fatigue, depression, weight gain), clonidine (Dixarit), and Bellergal, which contains phenobarbital, ergotamine, and belladonna (a *real* witches' brew, eh?).

### Step 6. Break and enter . . .

• Some gynecologists recommend hysterectomy as a cure for hot flashes. This is malpractice, as your uterus doesn't cause hot flashes. The only conceivable benefit would be that, once your uterus is removed, you can take ERT/HRT without worry of cervical or uterine cancer.

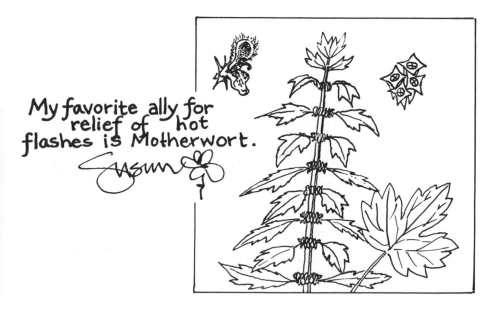

My favorite ally for relief of hot flashes is Motherwort.

# Night Sweats

### Step 1. Collect information . . .

A hot flash at night is called a night sweat. Night sweats may be accompanied or preceded by feelings of anxiety or terror. Some women have no night sweats, only daytime hot flashes; some women flash only at night and hardly at all during the day; most women get a chance to experience both.

### Step 2. Engage the energy . . .

• Try homeopathic *Nux vomica* when night sweats or leg cramps wake you and leave you feeling chilled and irritable.

• Try homeopathic *Sulfur* when whole-body night sweats leave you with a huge thirst and intolerance to heat in any form.

### Step 3. Nourish and tonify . . .

★ **Prepare your bed** to help.moderate hot flashes in your sleep. Use all-cotton sheets. Use a mattress of natural fibers (a futon is fine). Try a feather pillow. Perhaps a silk nightgown? The usual polyester blend sheets, foam rubber mattresses/pillows, and nylon sleeping wear encourage flashes and keep you damp and clammy afterward.

★ **Oatstraw** infusion, a cup or more a day, strengthens adrenals, promotes sound sleep, and reduces night sweats.

★ My favorite remedy for women disturbed by night sweats? **Motherwort!** Use 10-25 drops up to three times a day, or upon awakening with a night sweat. Expect results in two to four weeks.

### Step 4. Sedate/Stimulate . . .

★ **Garden sage** (*Salvia officinalis*) is renowned for its ability to reduce and eliminate night sweats. The effect is quite prompt, usually noticeable in a few hours, and long-lived, sometimes up to two days from a single cup of tea. For best results, make a sage infusion and drink it by diluting 1-4 tablespoons/20-60 ml of the infusion in a cup of hot or cold water.

*Steps 5 and 6* . . . see steps 5b and 6 under "Hot Flashes," page 66.

*"I started flashing at 47. This peaked the year after my periods stopped, at 54, with hourly flushes waking me in a sweat. They've tapered off in the four years since. I did have a flash this morning, but the last one was three days ago."*

# Earthquake Flashes

### Step 1. Collect information . . .

"Earthquake" or "volcano" flashes are to a normal flash as a tidal wave is to a normal tide: uncontrollable and devastating.

Earthquake flashes are rare and infrequent in women achieving menopause naturally. They are quite common among women who achieve menopause by surgery, chemotherapy, or radiation.

### Step 2. Engage the energy . . .

• Try homeopathic *Sulfur* for earthquake flashes accompanied by profuse sweating (which may smell strong) and where the flashes cover hands and feet as well as face and torso.

• Homeopathic *Crotalus* helps the woman with earthquake flashes accompanied by headaches, flooding, restlessness, or/and weakness; worse after sleep.

### Step 3. Nourish and tonify . . .

★ **Black cohosh** root tincture, 30-60 drops taken up to four times daily, is as effective in relieving severe hot flashes as ERT.

• **Motherwort** tincture, 25-40 drops taken every 4 hours while awake, is a tremendous ally for the woman whose earthquakes include emotional uproar, erratic heart beats, and palpitations.

• **Ginseng** (2 grams daily) and lots of jogging put an end to one woman's earthquake flashes following surgery.

• **Royal jelly**, the substance bees feed the larva destined to be the queen bee, has an almost mythic reputation for relieving earthquake flashing. Buy it in small glass ampules in Chinatown or your health food store. Dose is 3-7 ampules per week. If you find ampules containing royal jelly and ginseng, so much the better.

### Step 4. Sedate/Stimulate . . .

• Sucking on a piece of **hard candy** can head off a hot flash or moderate an earthquake flash.

### Step 5a & 5b. Use supplements; Use drugs . . .

• Women with earthquake flashes may take ERT believing it is more effective than anything else. But vitamin E seems equally effective in relieving severe hot flashes (and decreasing death from heart disease). For earthquake flashes, try very high doses, 800-1200 IU daily. Look for noticeable effects within ten days. (See vitamin E cautions, page 62.)

*Step 6. Break and enter . . .*

★ After surgical (or chemical) induction of menopause, use **vitex** berry tincture, 30-90 drops daily for thirteen months. This may not eliminate all hot flashes, but will moderate their severity and duration.

## Other Overheated Conditions:
### Dizziness, Dry Eyes, Burning Mouth, Formication

*Step 1. Collect information . . .*

As if flushing and flashing and sweating and chilling weren't difficult enough to learn to endure (even enjoy) on our menopausal journey, some women also experience a variety of other problems with or apart from their hot flashes: faintness, dizziness, a sick feeling, dry eyes, burning mouth, and formication (from the Latin word for ant, *formica*) — a prickly sensation as if ants were crawling over the skin.

These problems are all related to an overworked and "overheated" liver. In Traditional Chinese Medicine (TCM), the liver controls the smooth flow of energy in the body; if the liver is overworked, as it may well be during the menopausal years, too much energy can go to the head, resulting in dizziness, faintness, and headaches.

That inner "sick" feeling usually centers in the stomach area, just under the ribs, in the chakra called the solar plexus, ruled by (how did you know?) the liver.

Lack of vitamin A (produced in the liver from carotenes) results in loss of night vision. In TCM, the eyes are the opening to the liver. Dry eyes are related to an overworked, overheated liver.

Many medical systems have noted that the mouth and tongue manifest the general state of health of the whole person. A burning mouth suggests not only a "hot" liver but someone whose whole system is on overload. This woman is burning to say something, as well.

If the nerve-endings in your skin seem hypersensitive (even worse than the princess who felt the pea under all those mattresses), that's a sign of liver distress, too.

Note that dizziness may also be from hyperventilation (a by-product of anxiety, fatigue, and stress), reduced blood flow to the brain, or inner ear debris (more common with age). Regular exercise or hatha yoga can prevent and relieve these problems.

*Step 2. Engage the energy . . .*

• *Caladium* is the homeopathic remedy for creepy crawly itchy skin, aggravated by heat and worse at night. So is *Rhus tox.*

- The smell of **lavender oil** is said to relieve dizziness.

- The smell of **cedar** soothes the liver, reduces "touchiness."

- For dry eyes: place **quartz crystals** or cucumber slices or steeped chamomile tea bags on closed eyelids and imagine crying the tears of the earth. Try homeopathic *Berberis vulgaris*.

- Homeopathic *Thuja* or *Rhus tox.* are remedies for burning mouth.

***Step 3. Nourish and tonify . . .***

★ Menopausal women with itchy, sensitive skin, light-headedness, hot eyes and mouth have found quick relief from 10-20 drops of liver-nourishing **dandelion root** tincture taken 1-3 times daily.

- **Lady's mantle** tea, very strong, and lots of it, tones the liver and helps eliminate itchy sensations following hot flashes.

★ Cool and soothe your eyes, mouth, skin, and liver from the inside out with **oatstraw** infusions and from the outside in with oatstraw baths.

★ A compress of fresh **chickweed** soothes the eyes and restores moisture. An eyewash of 2-5 drops calendula tincture in a palm full of warm water, used once a day, will also help restore needed moisture to the eyes if used repeatedly for several weeks.

***Step 4. Sedate/Stimulate . . .***

★ "For instant relief of formication," writes midwife Wonshé, "use **raw beets**. Eat them grated or juiced, three times in one day."

★ If you have crawlingly sensitive skin that prevents sleep, reach for the **skullcap** tincture. Try 3-5 drops; repeat twice if needed. Tincture of the fresh flowering tops of **St. Joan's wort**, 25-30 drops, can be used with, or instead of, skullcap.

- Relieve burning mouth with a rinse of **calendula** blossom tincture, a dropperful diluted in a small amount of water.

- Drink a cup of **primrose** (*Primula*) flower tea when you feel nervous and faint, with a sick sensation. (See caution, page 97.)

- When you feel dizzy, breathe into your cupped hands, exhaling as slowly as you can.

***Step 5b. Use drugs . . .***

- Alcohol and prescription medications can dry your eyes, make your skin sensitive, dilate your blood vessels and diminish the blood supply to your brain, making you dizzy, all without a hot flash. (They aren't nice to your liver, either.)

# Emotional Uproar

*"Dear woman," sighs Grandmother Growth tenderly. "I see that Change has thinned the protective layers hiding your anger, your fears, your grief. Yes, I see your hidden feelings and secret desires exposed a little more with each hot flash. You may think your feelings are out of proportion, too sharp, quite insane. But, I assure you, they are only raw from neglect. Receive them without judgment, nourish them, and your 'uncontrollable' feelings during the menopausal years will lead you to the deepest heart of your own secrets.*

*"If you cannot tolerate those about you, leave. You are called to isolation. Go to the sheltering space of your Crone's Year Away.*

*"If you feel called by death, do not mistake this as a call to take your own life. It is a call to embrace your eventual death as fully as possible while living as fully as possible.*

*"You have given life. You have given life even if you have not had a child, my child; for you have given the gift of potential life to yourself and your people. Giving life is good in your culture.*

*"Now you leave behind this Mother aspect and take on your identity as Crone. The Crone gives death, knows death, honors the gift of death, feels the truth of death. But death is fearful, bad in your culture. As a baby Crone, you need to acknowledge the facts of life, one of which is that the mate and lover of life is death. Facing one's own death, whether real or symbolic, is an emotionally intense experience. Accepting the death-giving aspect of yourself in the face of your cultural disapproval is an act of great courage.*

*"Come, dear one, and join the dance of feeling, life, and death. Do a crazy Crone step, whirling around the emotional roller coaster; it's part of the journey to 'crazy old lady,' she who can act totally outside the social norms, who can recognize and use the complete and awesome power of her emotions."*

We all connect the turbulent hormones of adolescence with the turbulent emotions of young adulthood, and the hormonal changes of pregnancy with the intense emotions of motherhood. Just so, the flashing, flooding hormones of menopause precipitate flashing, flooding emotions in the "pubescent Crone."

With her menstrual moon tides ebbing, then flowing in unpredictable floods, her body sometimes suddenly drenched in sweat, and sleep elusive, how could her emotions remain untouched? Menopause is the classic time in our culture for women to go "crazy." Oversensitivity, irritability, anxiety, fear, extreme nervousness, rage, grief, depression, and crying jags are not uncommon during the menopausal climax years.

The remedies here don't seek to eliminate these emotions, or turn "negative" ones into "positive" ones, but, in the Wise Woman way, to help you incorporate all of your feelings into your wholeness.

*"In the midst of a hot flash, I suddenly saw my entire life in a new light. I wanted to rage; I wanted to laugh without stopping. I was afraid I was crazy, but I knew I'd never been more sane."*

# Depression

*"Look here," signals Grandmother Growth, spreading out a story blanket. "See how depression is deeply woven with anger and grief. When our human need for reliable, joyous intimacy is frustrated, and expression of our frustration would endanger us, depression comes and protects. When there is no way to deal effectively with situations that enrage us, depression comes and helps us still the violent impulse.*

*"Depression is not an easy companion on your journey, but let her go with us for a while. She knows much about life, about your life, and about the give-away of life and death. In her bundle, she carries the anger you have carefully frozen with frigid blasts of fear and kept nourished with your pain. Dare to accept her bundle, to accept your own wholeness. Dare to forgive what hurt you and stop reliving the pain. Dare to thaw your rage. You will need it, daughter, in the days to come."*

### Step 0. Do nothing . . .

• Welcome the dark. Cherish the deepness. Give yourself over to a day or two of doing nothing.

★ Return to earth. Go into your (metaphorical) cave. Lie belly down on the earth. Bury yourself in leaves or sand.

### Step 1. Collect information . . .

Depression is very common among women with induced menopause. But it is no more common among women achieving menopause naturally than among, say, single mothers. Why is it so associated with menopause in our minds and stories?

Depression can indicate hypothyroidism. Depression can be caused by steroids, high blood pressure drugs, and ERT/HRT. But most often the cause of depression is the belief (valid or not) that nothing you do makes any difference.

Victimization is one of the most significant risk factors in the development of depression; it is estimated that at least 40 percent of all women in the United States have been sexually or physically victimized. Poverty is also a precipitator of depression; women make up more than two-thirds of all Americans who live below poverty level. More than menopause, victimization and poverty put women of all ages at risk for depression and show clearly how depression is a "lid" on rage and pain.

**Get help if you are depressed for more than two weeks.** Call your local hot line; the number is in the front of your phone book. Or see page 88 for ways to contact feminist therapists.

These remedies are helpful for "ordinary" depression as well as the more severe "clinical" depression.

*Step 2. Engage the energy . . .*

★ Anger is part of depression. **Find your anger**; cherish it. (See "Rage," page 78.)

★ Taken together, the **Bach flower remedies**, *Wild Rose, Larch, Mustard, Gorse*, and *Gentian* help alleviate feelings of apathy, resignation, despondency, inferiority, despair, hopelessness, discouragement, self-doubt, and intense descending gloom.

• **Homeopathic remedies for depression:**
☞ *Arum metallicum*: with frequent thoughts of suicide, feels cut off from love and joy.
☞ *Sepia*: just wants to be left alone, disinterested in sex, and snaps angrily at her family and friends.
☞ *Calms Forte* (a blend including calcium): depression with crying.

• Let **sunlight** be your remedy. It's more than idle chatter that we identify depression with grey skies and happiness with sunny ones. Our hormonal/emotional balance is profoundly affected by sunlight. For emotional health (and strong bones) get 15 minutes of sunlight on your uncovered eyelids (take out contact lenses) daily. If you can't get out (or the sun doesn't cooperate) try sitting next to six to eight regular fluorescent tubes (2,500 lux) for thirty minutes each day upon waking.

★ **Sing the blues**; dance 'em, too. Women have depended on songs and dances to carry them out of depression for centuries. If you don't know how, sing along with Rosetta Records, page 88.

• **Dance therapy** or **massage therapy** is more effective than talk therapy for reaching and healing hidden traumas and relieving depression. Even a single session may have a dramatic effect.

- Aromatherapists suggest the smell of **lemon balm** (*Melissa*) tea or oil to lift spirits and ease depression.

- Menopause is an ideal time to renew your relationship with your maiden self, your **inner child**. As we embrace our past and bless it, depression lifts and the future smiles. (See "Inner Child Workbook".)

- Write in a journal. Talk to a friend.

### Step 3. Nourish and tonify . . .

★ **St. Joan's wort**, Johannaskraut, Herbe de la St. Jean (*Hypericum perforatum*) is mistakenly cited in many herbals as contraindicated for depression. Nothing could be further from the truth. I have repeatedly seen women relieve all types of depression, including SAD (seasonal affective disorder), and physical pains associated with depression, using 25 drops of the fresh flower tincture 1-3 times a day for several months.

★ Adrenal exhaustion gives rise to depression, fatigue, irritability, and unpredictable mood swings. Your adrenals expend a lot of extra energy making hormones during your menopausal years. Give them tender loving care with **nettle** infusion, 1-3 cups/250-750 ml daily.

★ **Oatstraw** infusion has been suggested for hysterical and depressed women since earliest times. Gentle *Avena* nourishes the nerves and helps you remember why life is worth living. Drink as many cups a day as you wish.

- **Garden Sage** (*Salvia*) is an ancient ally for emotionally distressed mid-life women. In some societies, only crones were allowed to drink the brew made from the nubbly leaves (at least partly because it delays menses and dries up breast milk). Make a quart/liter of the infusion. Dilute it to taste with hot water or warm milk and honey as you drink it. It will keep for weeks refrigerated; and leftovers make a great hair rinse.

★ **Walk and sing!**

★ Short-term cognitive behavioral therapy or interpersonal therapy has been clinically verified to be as effective as drugs in relieving depression. Not only that, two-thirds of those who simply read about therapy improved significantly.

★ **Thirty minutes of aerobic exercise**, especially soon after awakening, has been shown to relieve depressions resistant to all other treatments, including drugs.

*Step 4. Stimulate/Sedate . . .*

★ **Sleep less.** While we sleep, a depression-causing substance is produced and used. We usually awaken when we've used all we produced that night. Depressed women overproduce this substance while asleep and find it difficult to wake up. Going back to sleep compounds the problem. Staying up all night once a week can cure your depression. If you can't cope with no sleep, even mild sleep deprivation (such as sleeping five hours or less for two nights in a row) decreases depressive symptoms in some people dramatically.

★ **Imitate joy.** Stand tall, smile with your whole face (mouth, cheeks, eyes), and breathe deeply. You will either actually start feeling happier or make your rage/grief more visible and more easily accessed.

• To **energize** yourself when depressed: 1) sigh deeply many times, 2) hold your arms out in front of you for several minutes, 3) bounce up and down on the balls of your feet.

*Step 5a. Use supplements . . .*

• Increasing the amount of **vitamin B complex** in your diet with whole grains and supplements of up to 50 mg daily can ease depression.

• Low levels of **calcium** and **zinc** in the blood are frequently associated with depression. Supplements of up to 20 mg zinc and 1500 mg calcium are suggested.

*Step 5b. Use drugs . . .*

• Depression can be a side effect of estrogen/progestine therapy (HRT) as well as estrogen therapy (ERT). It is wise to avoid hormonal replacements if you already feel depressed during your menopausal years. Two studies assessing the effectiveness of ERT on menopausal depression found ERT ineffective in improving women's mental states, but strongly associated with an increase in suicide attempts.

• Antidepressant drugs are used frequently to relieve (control) menopausal women's feelings. But adverse reactions to antidepressant drugs are quite frequent in women (much more so than in men). CAUTION: Fatal toxic interactions can occur if you take Prozac (fluoxetine) with any of these: lithium, tricyclic antidepressants (Tofranil/imipramine, Elavil/amitriptyline, Norpramin/desipramine), or monoamine oxidase inhibitors (Nardil/phenelizine, Parnate/tranylcypromine).

• Women taking lithium can gradually switch over to skullcap (*Scutellaria lateriflora*) infusion or tincture. Try 5-8 drops of fresh flowering plant tincture up to four times a day, or infusion of the dried plant, a cup/250 ml or more a day.

### Step 6. Break and enter . . .

• Medicine is not so quick these days to take menopausal women from their homes and lock them away. Drugs have virtually replaced locked institutions and shock therapy. Now women are locked away in their own minds and not allowed to come out until we can think "straight." The crazy Crone breaks all the rules; she jimmies all the locks.

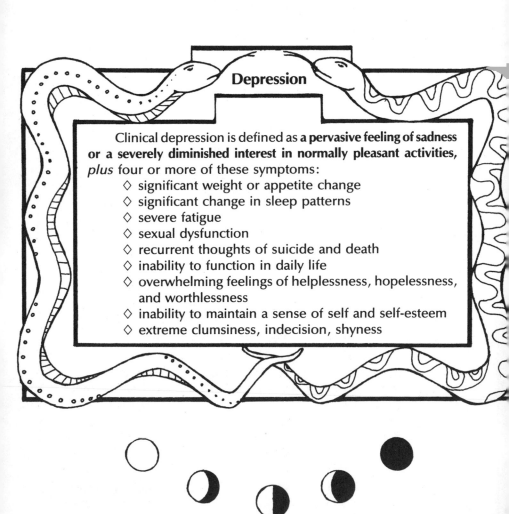

**Depression**

Clinical depression is defined as **a pervasive feeling of sadness or a severely diminished interest in normally pleasant activities,** *plus* four or more of these symptoms:
◊ significant weight or appetite change
◊ significant change in sleep patterns
◊ severe fatigue
◊ sexual dysfunction
◊ recurrent thoughts of suicide and death
◊ inability to function in daily life
◊ overwhelming feelings of helplessness, hopelessness, and worthlessness
◊ inability to maintain a sense of self and self-esteem
◊ extreme clumsiness, indecision, shyness

# Thoughts of Suicide

Like uncontrollable emotions, thoughts of suicide are normal for menopausal women. Remember that the death phase of this menopausal initiation does not imply actual physical death. Yet it would be foolish to deny that the *feeling* of dying can be as real as if it were actually happening.

There is a physical/emotional logic to thoughts of suicide. These rightly disturbing thoughts can show the menopausal woman the next steps on her journey. Real suicide is an act of desperate self-empowerment. But thoughts of suicide can be pathways to wholeness, health, and self-realization. Like depression, suicidal thoughts during menopause are potent guides to truth and joy.

Explore the logic of your suicide thought. What is its gift? How can you receive it without harming yourself? Suppose you want to take a flying leap. Jumping off a high place gives an intense experience of falling, flying, being free of restraint, unsupported, giving in to gravity. What other means are available to achieve these feelings? The answer may be as simple as learning to stand on your head in yoga, or as complex as doing something you've never done, never thought you could do: something exciting, terrifying, such as going on vacation totally by yourself, taking flying lessons, learning to ski, or trekking in the Himalayas.

If you feel like taking a gun to your head, you may need to learn to open the crown chakra. If you'd like to end it all by taking pills and passing out, you may need to admit to your exhaustion and take a rest. If you were to cut your wrists (cut off your hands, symbolically), what would you no longer have to put your hands to?

If you feel compelled to actually hurt yourself, do call the local crisis hot line listed in the front of your phone book. As with any decision about health, a wise woman seeks a second opinion.

*"My experience is that when a woman's estrogen levels get really low, she'll wake up suddenly in the middle of the night feeling suicidal, and she can't understand it. Let women know this is common and others experience it. Nourishing, estrogen-enhancing herbs [like black cohosh or sage] offer relief."*                                                           —Holly Eagle

# Rage

*With a great grin, Grandmother Growth winks and confides: "The self-initiated Crone is an outrageous hag. In order to be outrageous, you must contact and own your rage. Focused anger is the same energy as the uterine contractions of birth and menstruation: it pushes; it is hard. Give your anger a sturdy obstacle to push against; let it move outward. Anger focused outward with Crone wisdom has changed, and will continue to change, the courses of nations. Beware of hiding your anger, of focusing it inward; this brings resentment, spite, sulkiness, depression, death of the community, and fantasies of self-destruction."*

**Step 1. Collect information . . .**

Anger makes your heart pound, your palms sweat, and your blood pressure rise. Anger doesn't cause disease. Repressing it does, increasing rates of heart disease and cancer in women and doubling our mortality.

Menopausal women are described as irrational, ill-tempered, out of control, and insane when we speak the angry truth about our individual and collective lives in women-hating societies. To maintain the current social order, the rage of mature women must be disparaged and silenced. Unheard, unseen, unable to create the **Change** we envision, we turn our rage inward, we internalize social hatred toward women and naturally think of suicide. Why not, instead, be mad enough to live?

**Step 2. Engage the energy . . .**

★ *Cherry plum* is the **Bach flower remedy** for menopausal women about to do something desperate. It is suggested for those moments when you're afraid your anger is almost out of control, when you're on the verge of mental collapse, or when you're obsessed with thoughts of doing terrible things. Take 1-4 drops of the remedy frequently, under your tongue, while you ask yourself: Is there some way to achieve my vision other than this desperate action? ("I want to kill my mate. Then I would be alone. Hmmm . . . How about a vacation? Alone!") If you don't have cherry plum, use *Rescue Remedy.* If you don't have that, put some water in a special glass and use that as your remedy.

• Homeopathic *Lachesis* is suggested for the menopausal woman whose rage is evidenced by outbursts of irrational jealousy.

• Read "The Dance of Anger." Read "Kali: The Feminine Force." (See References & Resources, page 88.)

• Do the Kundalini Meditation. (See pages 60-61.)

*Step 3. Nourish and tonify . . .*

• Try the "NO!" remedy on pages 136-7.

• **Twist** a towel and growl; you can bite it, too. Grrr . . .

• **Hit** a hard object (like a wooden chair) with a rolled up newspaper or use Elisabeth Kübler-Ross's favorite, a length of rubber radiator hose and a big city phone directory or two. Start with inarticulate sounds. Gradually add short, simple phrases such as "No!" or "I'm furious!" IMPORTANT: Stay in the present and prevent dizziness while doing this by keeping your eyes open and focused. Pick a point on the floor or wall and concentrate on it, stare at it. Let the fire in your eyes come through. See if you can burn a hole in the wall with your gaze.

• Take time to be gentle with yourself after feeling rage, especially if rage is a new ally for you. Go for a walk, rearrange the bookshelf, listen to music, draw.

*Step 4. Sedate/Stimulate . . .*

★ With thanks to my teacher Gay Luce, I offer you the **temper tantrum** in a small space, for those times when you must have a raging fit but it just won't do to have it in public. To start, find a toilet stall, closet, or other small private space; you will need a little room to move. Then disorient yourself by shaking, everything, energetically: arms, legs, lips, eyes, fingers, head, toes, shoulders, all at once and without rhythm. Continue for at least a minute. Then inhale massively and hold your breath while you stamp your feet and strike out with your hands. If you really have to be quiet, you can sit on the toilet and kick with your feet, instead of stamping. If you can make some noise, let a sound come out when you finally stop and exhale. If I really put energy into the disorientation, one tantrum is usually enough; you may need to do it 2-3 times at first. And one more hint: practice this before you really need to use it.

• The color **pink** relaxes muscles in seconds. Pink rooms are currently used quite successfully in prisons to calm hostile, aggressive inmates.

*Step 5b. Use drugs . . .*

• **Tranquilizers** will end that terrible feeling of wanting to destroy everything. So will sugar and alcohol. But it only *seems* easier to destroy ourselves rather than put an end to that which enrages us. The Crone's rage keeps her community alive with conscience, truth, and beauty. (See pages 84-85 for warnings on uses of tranquilizers.)

*Step 6. Break and enter . . .*

• Go ahead and break something. The sound of shattering glass sings the truth of rage. Go to your local recycling center and see if you can safely break glass there. One friend has a special set of dishes and a special (safe) place to break them when she's "uncontrollably enraged."

# Grief/Crying Jags

*"Gone are the days when you wept uncontrollably one day and found yourself bleeding the next. Now you cry and there's no blood the next day. So you cry; and cry. Love your tears, Crone-to-be," croons Grandmother Growth. "Feel the grief of life, the grief of death. Let these tears flood your heart with compassion.*

*"Grieve all that is lost to you, dear one. Grieve all potential that never thrived. Grieve the beauty extinguished too soon. Grieve the wounds of all women, all souls.*

*"Grief is an important part of your self-initiation as Crone, great granddaughter. As a menopausal woman you are watching the death of yourself as fertile Mother-woman. So it is fair to cry, to weep, and grieve. Come, cry here on my shoulder."*

*Step 0. Do nothing . . .*

• When the grief is deep and mourning is fully engaged in, sobbing will sound hysterical (that is, as though coming from the womb/belly). This will stop when exhaustion sets in, rarely before. Go to bed. Be patient. Love yourself.

*Step 1. Collect information . . .*

Denied and restricted, grief contracts the muscles, especially those of the throat and chest. Allowed, grief can throb through your body and soul in deep, loose, primal sobs; then tenderly and softly push you, birth you, into vital and vibrant new life.

*Step 2. Engage the energy . . .*

• The Bach flower remedy *Mustard* is advised for those in deep gloom.

• Grief likes to cling, to hold on; so hold on to something soft and plush. And if it is a fat pillow stuffed with hops (soothing) or lavender (sweetening) or sage (transforming), all the better.

• What rituals of mourning have you participated in? What rituals of mourning have you read about? Create a ritual of mourning for yourself, just exactly as you would like it.

*Step 3. Nourish and tonify . . .*

★ **Motherwort**, tincture of the fresh plant in flower, 10-15 drops, 2-3 times a day for several weeks, mellows the sharpness of grief.

★ **Passion flower** herb (*Passiflora*) is used wherever it grows to treat all types of hysteria. (Hysteria, by the way, refers to feelings from the womb, which is *hystera* in Greek.) Try it if your crying brings on a headache or leaves you twitchy and restless. A dose of the tincture of the fresh plant in flower is 10-25 drops as needed.

• **Lemon balm** (*Melissa*) is a soothing friend to a crying woman. Brew a tea of the fresh leaves and drink freely.

• **Ginseng** and **Dong Quai/Dang Gui** roots can help you deal with stress. Chew either one or take in tincture form, up to 30 drops a day.

*Step 4. Sedate/Stimulate . . .*

• **Hops** tea offers you lots of B vitamins (depleted when fluids such as tears and sweat are lost from the body), a calming touch to the nerves, and plenty of hormones to even out the snags. Overindulgence may put you to sleep; and that may be just what you need.

★ When sobbing continues for days, muscles can get very sore. **St. Joan's wort** tincture relieves and prevents such soreness. A dose of 25 drops (up to 6 times a day) prevents and eliminates lactic acid build-up in the muscles, deepens sleep, eases depression, and strengthens the nerves.

*Step 5a. Use supplements . . .*

★ Large doses of B vitamin complex for several days can dramatically improve your ability to handle the stress of grief.

*Step 5b. Use drugs . . .*

• Tranquilizers, again? See pages 84-85.

# Anxiety/Fear/Extreme Nervousness

*"Have you noticed?" whispers Grandmother Growth. "Your hot flushes and menstrual irregularities disrupt your normal patterns, make openings for your buried fears to emerge. Welcome these fears; they bring memories. Memories of childhood, memories of other lives. Often these memories find easiest access to your consciousness through fear. If you reject your fear, it will immobilize you, shorten your breath, leave you speechless, and dim your full delight in life. Approach with curiosity; let your fear bring you gifts of self-awareness. (Note how dilated the pupils become*

*in fear: anxious eyes take in everything.) Hold my hand. Say 'I'm afraid.'
And take a step forward."*

### Step 1. Collect information . . .

Adrenal energy is associated with fear; adrenalin is the "fight or flight" hormone. During menopause, when the adrenals take on the extra task of contributing estrogen/estrone to the hormonal dance, they can easily become depleted. The exhausted adrenals then over-react, giving rise to sudden sensations of anxiety, fear, and nervousness. For example, the need to make a minor decision can cause a surge of adrenalin, triggering a hot flash and leaving you feeling mentally blank, physically wiped out, anxious, and fearful of what's happening to you.

### Step 2. Engage the energy . . .

★ Try these **Bach flower remedies**, 1-4 drops at a time, as needed:
☞ *Aspen*: fear of the unknown, apprehension, and anxiety.
☞ *Mimulus*: fear of the known.
☞ *Red Chestnut*: anxious and fearful for others' safety.
☞ *Elm*: overwhelmed and inadequate.
☞ *Rock Rose*: renowned for easing terror and panic.

• Aromatherapists suggests the smell of **rose** to ease anxiety and fears. Touch the essential oil to the seam of your sleeve and wrap youself in calming fragrance all day.

★ Even one session of **massage** can cause a marked decrease in anxiety and fearfulness. Add a few drops of **lavender** to your massage oil to induce even more tranquility.

★ Fear and anxiety give rise to hard, contracted muscles and shallow breathing. To **unfreeze** yourself, try curling up in a fetal position (on your side with knees drawn up), breathing deeply, and humming. Ummmm . . . . It's fine to rock back and forth, too. What feeling wants to emerge from the fear? Grief is soft, but still contracted. Rage is hard and will make you uncurl.

★ With the assistance of a friend, use **gentle touch** to restore your sense of calm. Lie on your stomach. Have your friend rest their right hand on your sacrum, fingers touching and pointing toward your head; their left is hand at your neck, fingers together and pointed toward the head. In silence, let the hands rest comfortably for 1-5 minutes.

★ **Claim your boundaries.** Anxiety arises when we feel unsafe. Where can you be safe? Who supports you in the full expression of your self/selves? Identify and create the physical, psychic, emotional bound-aries and rules you need in order to feel really safe.

• If you are overcome with unfocused anxiety, **focus** your eyes. Look at anything steadily while breathing deeply. Generate energy in your solar plexus.

• If your anxiety/nervousness is specifically focused, take all your worry-ing energy and use it to create a huge **image of safety** (like a cowrie shell, Buddha's or Christ's palm, a giant mother's lap). Surround the object of your anxiety with this image as often as necessary. Fear locks up movement and speech, yet any direct action, even mental, can unfreeze fear.

### Step 3. Nourish and tonify . . .

• How about a class in **self-defense**? There really are things to be afraid of; best to know how to deal with them.

★ Sister stinging **nettle** is the remedy of choice to nourish the adrenals and relieve anxiety. Brew a rich infusion and drink freely.

• When the worries go 'round and 'round in your brain, **talk** to someone who will listen in silence. No matter how stupid or silly your fears seem, express them out loud with a witness.

• **Nourish your fear. Fear and desire are not opposites; they're the same.** When I don't want to admit to myself what I want, I turn my desire into a fear so I can hold it close and keep it at a distance at the same time. What would your life be like if your fears came true?

• **Yoga** postures, yoga breathing, and quiet, focused meditation tonify (and soothe) the sympathetic nervous system. Regular practice alle-viates anxiety, often permanently.

• Try a dropperful (or two) of **St. Joan's wort** (*Hypericum*) tincture when you're on the edge and feeling like anything will push you over it. You can safely repeat the dose several times an hour if you wish. This nerve-nourishing and nerve-strengthening herb relieves the immediate anxiety and helps prevent future distress as well.

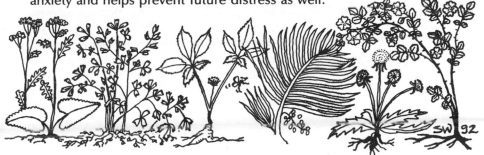

### Step 4. Sedate/Stimulate . . .

• Fear wants to pull in, contract; let the muscles relax in a **hot tub** or **sauna**. Ahhh . . . Or try a **lemon balm** bath; it's an ancient remedy for bad cases of the "nerves."

★ **Exercise** of any kind is often a ready remedy for overwhelming anxiety. Movement and fear don't coexist easily. If you feel like running away from it all, running might be the very thing to do. Fifteen to twenty minutes of heart-pounding exercise will use up your excess adrenalin and "eat up" your stress.

★ If you feel so anxious you think you might burst and do crazy things, try the **lion pose**. Open your mouth very wide; even wider. Stick your tongue out; even further. Open your eyes really wide; bigger. Rotate eyes left, then right. Breathe deeply and exhale fully up to ten times. Keep the shoulders and the forehead relaxed. This pose unblocks the throat, releases facial tension, relaxes the breathing muscles, and relieves anxiety.

• Extreme fear or anxiety may lead to hyperventilation. If you are breathing rapidly and shallowly and feel spaced out you can 1) breathe into a paper bag until normal breathing resumes or 2) hold your breath (you can actually put your hand over your nose and mouth) for a count of 20; then breathe out as slowly as you can.

• Reach for **skullcap** or **motherwort**, 8-10 drops of the fresh plant tincture, taken in some water, to steady your nerves and calm your thoughts.

• **Valerian** is the herbal tranquilizer. Try tiny five-drop doses of the fresh root tincture, but repeat every 10-15 minutes until you are calm. Use for no more than three weeks at a time.

### Step 5a. Use supplements . . .

★ **Calcium** supplements, up to 1500 mg a day, help relieve anxiety. (See page 26.)

### Step 5b. Use drugs . . .

★ **Tranquilizers** are more commonly prescribed for menopausal women than estrogen. There's even a brand of ERT (Menrium) with a tranquilizing drug included. Tranquilizers are dangerous to menopausal women.

☞ Prescription tranquilizers are addictive, and anyone taking them risks addiction. Sudden withdrawal causes severe symptoms, including seizures. Slower withdrawal causes the very distresses the tranquilizer was supposed to cure: anxiety, restlessness, sleep disturbances, headaches, shaking, visual disturbances, and a generally "yuck" feeling.

☞ The majority of women taking tranquilizers feel drowsy all day. Many also have side effects such as dizziness, decreased coordination, slowed reaction times, inability to concentrate or read a book, and decreased mental functioning, including memory loss, learning blocks, and confusion. One MD states: "Three-quarters of the patients I see who take Librium or Valium in normal doses have impaired intellectual functions."

☞ The risk of breaking a bone is five times greater than usual among those taking tranquilizers; and the effect continues for three or more months after taking the last one. Most people on tranquilizers don't realize how shaky on their feet and slow to react they've become.

★ If a chemical tranquilizer/sleeping pill *is* chosen, the advice of Sidney Wolfe, MD, is to use 7.5 milligrams (½ of a tablet) of oxazepam (Serax) for no more than seven days. Have the doctor write NO REFILL on the scrip. Do not drink any alcohol. Do try at least one remedy from step 2 and one from step 3 at the same time.

**Step 6. Break and enter . . .**

★ Suicide has been linked to regular use of tranquilizers, as have nightmares, sleep disturbances, and depression.

★ In an ironic twist, some women seem to discover their rage when dosed with tranquilizers.

# Oversensitivity/Irritability

*"If you would be Crone, dear woman, you will be as sensitive as I am,"* says Grandmother Growth from the shadows. *"My skin is sensitive; I feel the tiniest crinkle in my bed. My ears are sensitive; I seem to hear and understand the conversations of all life. My eyes are sensitive; I see exceptionally well at night. My nose and mouth are sensitive; I can find water by smelling, identify the uses of a plant by tasting. My emotional body is sensitive; I feel untruths as physical discomfort.*

*"Do not think of this sensitivity as a problem, a disability. Experience it as expansion, not limitation. Sensitivity isn't easy to live with; like nature, it doesn't tolerate sloppiness. In your civilized world, sensitivity may be a detriment, but in the natural world, sensitivity keeps you alive.*

*"Let us honor the heightened sensitivities of the Crones! Our communities depend on the Crones' irritability for their very survival. In their sensitivity, the Crones are irritated first by that which has the ability to poison all of us, whether it is a food, a feeling, or a rule."*

### Step 0. Do nothing . . .

• Is your oversensitivity a way to create some space around yourself? Is this Grandmother Growth's way of reminding you to take some time alone? It is OK to be antisocial. Dance by yourself. Stay home and read "Reinventing Eve" or "Circle of Stones."

### Step 1. Collect information . . .

PMS-like emotional sensitivity is aggravated during the menopausal years by sleepless nights, embarrassing hot flashes, and short-term memory loss. Nourishing the adrenals offers smoother emotional responses. Nourishing the nerves allows more energy to move with less friction. Nourishing the self-image encourages the emergence of the wise Crone.

### Step 2. Engage the energy . . .

★ The Bach flower remedy *Walnut* offers protection from outside influences. Use it as a buffer during the height of your menopausal sensitivity and as a guide when you encounter (or call up) symbolic death states. You can also carry a whole walnut in the shell for protection.

• The Bach flower remedy *Impatiens* helps when you feel irritable and impatient. Buy it or make a similiar remedy by floating the flowers from cultivated *Impatiens* or wild jewel weed (*Impatiens capensis*) in a bowl of spring or rain water for several hours in the sun. (Preserve by mixing with brandy, half and half.) Use 1-4 drops as often as desired.

### Step 3. Nourish and tonify . . .

★ **Oatstraw** gives the emerging crone amazing endurance. How easily irritability subsides when nerve energy flows smoothly. Drink oatstraw infusion freely. (The Bach flower remedy, *Wild Oat*, is for those seeking the true goal of their life.)

★ **Yoga**—not just the postures, but the breathing and focusing exercises as well—helps create strength in the nerves, adrenals, and heart, making sensitivity and irritability an ally rather than a liability.

• Oversensitivity is connected to the **liver** in several traditional healing theories. What's your local liver-loving weed? Dandelion, yellow dock, thistle? Find out. Make friends; invite her to dinner often.

### Step 4. Sedate/Stimulate . . .

★ Treat yourself to a full-body **massage**. It will relax your muscles so you can be at ease with your heightened sensitivity and it may awaken deadened places in your emotional body, as well.

★ **Skullcap** infusion or tincture strengthens the nerves and eases oversensitivity. I take 4-8 drops in some water in the morning if I want to be a little "tougher" emotionally; I take the same at night if I need to sleep deeply.

• Television, alcohol, and mindless games are common ways of numbing sensitivities. Substitute volunteer work, gardening, and exercise; they keep you just as occupied in the short run and improve health in the long run.

★ If you suddenly stop drinking coffee, you may feel hypersensitive. Lots of **water** (a glass every hour) helps calm the sensory overload.

*Step 5a. Use supplements . . .*

★ **Calcium** supplements, 250-500 mg a day, help calm the most jangled nerves.

*Step 5b. Use drugs . . .*

• Tranquilizers are frequently prescribed for menopausal women who are too "uppity." See pages 84-85.

*Step 6. Break and enter . . .*

★ Being **buried** for 8-24 hours in sand or earth (with face exposed) and left alone is a dramatic way to transform your feelings of extreme sensitivity. I have found this "primitive psychotherapy"—which involves a real, yet symbolic, statement of the underlying assumption ("I don't want to feel anything") — to be incredibly effective in helping the individual integrate and contact a rich wholeness/healthiness.

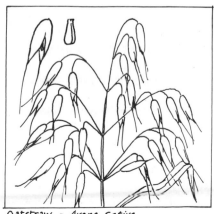

Oatstraw - *Avena Sativa*

## Emotional Uproar
# References & Resources

American Dance Therapy Association, 2000 Century Plaza, Suite 108, Columbia, MD 21044

Anger workshop materials from Institute for Mental Health Initiatives, 4545 42nd Street NW, Suite 311, Washington, DC, 20016

Association for Women in Psychology, Ellyn Kaschak, Dept of Psychology, San Jose State, San Jose, CA 95192 • List of feminist therapists.

"Circle of Stones: Woman's Journey to Herself," Judith Dnerk, Lura Media, 1989. $6 from 7060 Miramar Rd., Suite 104, San Diego, CA 92121

"Control Your Depression," P. Lewisohn, Prentice Hall, 1991 • Behavioral.

"Cries of the Spirit: A Celebration of Women's Spirituality," Marilyn Sewell, editor, Beacon, 1991

"Dance of Anger: A Woman's Guide," Harriet Lerner, Harper & Row, 1990

"Depression is a Feminist Issue," Beverly Burnside, 1990

"Depression: What Can Be Done?" Health Facts, Vol. XV, #128, Jan. 1990

"Emotional First Aid," Sean Haldane, Station Hill, 1989

"Feeling Good: The New Mood Therapy," DD Burns, NAL, 1990

Feminist Therapy Institute, Clare Holzman, 330 West 58th St, NY, NY 10019 (212) 245-7282

"Healing into Life and Death," Stephen Levine, Anchor/Doubleday, 1987 • On becoming whole through anger, grief, fear.

"How to Get Going When You Can Barely Get Out of Bed," Linda Bailey, Prentice Hall, 1984 • Practical advice and exercises.

"How Anger Affects Your Health," University of California at Berkeley Wellness Letter, January 1992

"Inner Child Workbook," Cathryn Taylor, Tarcher, 1991

"Kali: The Feminine Force," A. Mookerjee, Destiny, 1988

"Meeting the Shadow: The Hidden Power of the Dark Side of Human Nature," Connie Zweig & J. Abrams, editors, Tarcher, 1991

National Task Force on Depression, Director of Women's Programs, APA, 1200 Seventeenth St NW, Washington, DC 20036

Option Institute, RD1, Box 174A, Sheffield, MA 01257 • Feeling workshops.

"Pathwork of Self Transformation," Eva Pierrakos, Bantam, 1990 • Highly recommended, deep reading, deep work.

"Reinventing Eve," Kim Chernin, Harper, 1986

Rosetta Records, 115 W. 16th St, NY, NY 10011 • My favorite blues tapes.

Self Care Catalog, 5850 Shellmound Avenue, Emeryville, CA 94662-0813 • Mail order source for 2500 lux light fixtures.

Society for Light Treatment and Biological Rhythm, 722 West 168th St, Box 50, NY, NY 10032

Wise Woman Center, POBox 64, Woodstock, NY 12498 • Wise Woman workshops.

# Sleep Disturbances

*"Do you know the way to your dream time?" The voice of Grandmother Growth comes inside your ear, just as you thought you were falling asleep. "When you claim the transformation of menopause, you can enter dream time any time. When you hold your wise blood inside, dreams come at your bidding. So does sleep.*

*"But not just yet. Not until after you've journeyed with me into seeming chaos, into the sleepless, timeless, visionary place of the Crone. Much that has bound you, young Crone, will unravel in the nights to come. Your wisdom is waking. And so will you.*

*"You won't sleep well during the short part of your menopause when you may be swept by waves of volcanic heat, shiver through arctic chills, have sweat rivering through your bed clothes, and feel powerful surges of emotion. There may be times when your mind and hormones and memories make a crazy quilt of your dreams and days. Surely you wouldn't expect to sleep peacefully through that.*

*"Inspiration may shake you awake before dawn. Be ready to receive the gifts of this Change, whether awake or asleep. Be ready; what you thought were walls are veils," comes her voice, like the breeze, soft.*

**Step 0. Do nothing . . .**

• Relieve yourself of all responsibility for even a day or two (better a week or two) so you can be free to sleep whenever the mood strikes.

• Free yourself from the rule of time so you can catnap and tap into your creativity at any hour of the day or night. Put away all clocks and watches for a few days. Don't listen to the radio or ask for the time. Let the earth and moon and sun provide your timing.

**Step 1. Collect information . . .**

Sleep disturbances are a frequent, but generally short-lived, part of the menopausal **Change.** Some menopausal women sleep restlessly, wake early, go for a walk, need a nap later. Others feel so tense when they lie down they can't seem to drift off, and wake achy and irritated. A few menopausal women experience sleep disturbances for so many nights on end that they soon have the look of a new mother (of twins).

*"I was 40; my tubal ligation accidentally fried my ovaries. I'd go to sleep and wake up in a terrible sweat. I'd throw the covers off and open the window and go back to sleep. In 15 minutes I was frozen, awake again, covering up, dropping off to sleep, only to awaken 20 minutes later in a terrible sweat. I'd throw the covers off and open the window and go back to sleep. In 15 minutes I was frozen, awake again, and again, and again all night."*

*Step 2. Engage the energy . . .*

• Create a **bedtime routine**: go to bed at the same time each night, read for thirty minutes or listen to taped music, then go to sleep; if not asleep in thirty minutes, read or listen to more music for another half hour before going to sleep. (This is behavior modification; see step 5.)

★ **Keep a journal** by your bed. Creative juices flow wildly during menopause; if you're up when they are, grab 'em.

★ **Lavender blossoms** and their essential oil are crone classics; didn't your granny smell of lavender? The strong but agreeable odor brings sleep at night, relieves dizziness and faintness during the day. Sleep with a little pillow of lavender blossoms; slip it into your pocket when you dress. Or use a few drops of the essential oil on a handkerchief tucked into your pillow or purse. A lavender bath before bed (use a few drops of oil or a handful of dried flowers) eases the mind and body, and evokes soothing dreams.

★ No matter how little you sleep, you can feel energetic and refreshed if you **relax** deeply and completely. Visualizing or fantasizing is an ideal way to relax, often leading to sleep. (If other thoughts intrude, just return to your fantasy.) See box, page 91.

*Step 3. Nourish and tonify . . .*

★ Let **oatstraw** nourish your nervous system, smoothe your energy flow, and give you more restful sleep. Her cooling nourishing ways ease night sweats, anxiety, and headaches. Oatstraw is renowned for her antidepressant effect. Try a cup of infusion before bed, warm, with milk. And another at breakfast. Or try sleeping on an oat hull pillow. You can't overdose on bone-strengthening, gland-nurturing oatstraw; drink freely.

• **Hops** tea is a powerful sleep inducer and wonderful hormonal ally to the woman awakened frequently by night sweats. Keep a cup on the night stand to slip you back to sleep. A small pillow of dried hops blossoms under your head also helps entice sleep into your bed.

★ **Nettle,** nourisher of the energy circuits and the adrenals, isn't usually considered a sleep inducer. But it might be for you. Here's how. It is theorized that night sweats occur when the adrenals are triggered (usually by a sound) and flood the blood with adrenalin, which causes a hot flash. (Whether by the flash itself, the chill after, or the adrenalin-induced panic preceding, you are awakened.) Producing adrenalin stresses the adrenals, however. Every time this cycle occurs, the adrenals are stressed a little more and thus are more easily triggered by smaller and smaller sounds, resulting in more and more frequent sleep disruptions. Remedy: Nourish your adrenals with nettle infusion, a cup or more four times a week, and get some ear plugs (the little foam cylinder ones that you can buy for a quarter are great), and soon you'll sleep, sleep, sleep.

• Nerve-nourishing **St. Joan's wort** (*Hypericum*) tincture is also a gentle beckoner of sleep. Use a dropperful in a cup of fresh hops or lemon balm tea for a double dose of slumber.

## Susun's Favorite Relaxation

I am peacefully and happily lolling on a sandy beach listening to the waves. The wind and the sun and the shade touch me in just the right proportions.

The sound of the waves gets gradually louder as the tide comes in. The flowing waves lap over my toes and then recede. Slowly. I smell the tang of the brine as the waves cover my ankles, then pull down to my toes. Slowly, caressingly, the waves rise up to my knees, slide down my calves.

I hear and feel the waves as they reach up to my mid-thighs and pull back down to behind my knees. The waves rise and fall rhythmically; up to my hips, down my thighs. Content, at ease, I settle deeper into the sand as the warm water curls up and around me and pulls the sand away from underneath my back and buttocks.

The waves continue to spread over me, then pull away. The water covers my hips, my fingertips, my waist, my lower arms, my breasts, my shoulders.

I feel safe and secure as the moving water rocks me. I let the water come as high as I like. Sometimes it covers my face as I breathe out and slips away just before I breathe in. Sometimes I float. (Actually, I usually fall asleep before the water gets past my knees.)

### Step 4. Sedate/Stimulate . . .

★ Delicious, aromatic **skullcap** tincture is my favorite pain killer and sleep-inducer. Tincture of fresh flowering *Scutellaria lateriflora* even brings sleep to those addicted to sleeping pills. Though powerful, skullcap rarely leaves a muggy feeling next morning. Long-term use is not addictive, but rarely needed. Try 3-8 drops in a cup of water or herbal infusion about thirty minutes before lights out. Repeat at bedtime. (And once again in twenty minutes if needed.)

★ **Passion flower** herb, Passionskraut, Passiflore (*Passiflora incarnata*) is an old wives' remedy for nervous insomnia and hysteria, restlessness and headaches. With its unique, purple-crowned flowers, it visually says "crone." Try 15-60 drops of the fresh flowering plant tincture before bed each evening to relieve ongoing sleeplessness. (Note: Passion fruits are a rich source of estrogenic bioflavonoids.)

• Tincture of the fresh root of **valerian**, Baldrian, Valériane (*Valeriana officinalis*) is one of the most powerful plant sedatives known. Highly regarded as an ally for women pained by menstrual cramps, valerian is also a friend to the menopausal woman who's desperate for a night's sleep. Valerian also helps resolve chronic headaches (even migraines), decreases anxiety, and reduces fatigue. Use 20-30 drops just before bed; repeat in thirty minutes if needed. CAUTION: Valerian can be as habit-forming as some drugs if used nightly.

• Coffee, black tea, or alcohol contribute to night sweats and unrestful, agitated sleep. For some menopausal women, these stimulants prevent sleep altogether and trigger intense hot flashes.

### Step 5a. Use supplements . . .

• Try 500 mg **calcium** at bedtime for a sound night's sleep.

• CAUTION: Amino acids in pill form are synthetic drugs, not natural substances. Yes, L-tryptophan helps induce sleep, but it is not identical to the naturally occurring R-tryptophan found in foods.

### Step 5b. Use drugs . . .

• Sleep-inducing drugs are habit-forming. The ones most commonly prescribed are benzodiazepines such as Valium, Xanax, Dalmane, Doral, Halcion, ProSom, and Restoril. Side effects of benzodiazepines include next-day memory loss, confusion, anxiety, and excitability. Considering their stressful effects on the nervous system, these drugs seem entirely inappropriate for the sleep-deprived menopausal woman. To avoid the worst side effects of these drugs, take them for no more than 2-3 weeks and at half the usual dose.

★ Behavior modification therapy has been shown to be four times more effective than drugs in reducing the time needed to fall asleep and in increasing the actual span of restful sleep. (See step 2.)

### Step 6. Break and enter . . .

"Sleep deprivation has been a very powerful tool for me in breaking down my control barriers and making way for the information that the universe wants me to have. In my opinion, sleep deprivation is more powerful than most psychoactive drugs."

# Fatigue

*"Fall into my arms and sleep," offers Grandmother Growth. "You don't have to make this change happen; it will happen on its own. Let me hold you. Let go. Don't resist. Rest. You are in the midst of the labor of giving birth to yourself as Crone. Of course you are tired. This is hard work.*

*"Let the pushing energy of your uterus move your energy up to your crown, rather than down and out, as with menstrual blood and babies. This birthing of your wholeness is something you'll retain, not something you'll birth and give away. Rest in my strong arms. Take courage. "*

### Step 0. Do nothing . . .

• Extreme fatigue during menopause indicates a profound need to do nothing. Take a Crone's Time Away or at least arrange a short time-out.

• Give yourself a "well day" before you have to take a sick day. Ask family and friends to give you a day totally off . . . and take it! Barricade yourself in your room if need be (or, like the cartoon character Sylvia, in the bathroom).

### Step 1. Collect information . . .

Internal processes occurring during menopause demand tremendous amounts of energy, leaving a deficit for your external life unless you provide yourself with very high quality nutrients and use your energy wisely.

Women whose menopause is induced generally experience more extreme fatigue than women who achieve menopause naturally. And women whose sleep is disrupted with frequent night sweats frequently feel worn out and tired all day. Even if you achieve menopause naturally and are resting well, you may have less energy for things outside yourself during the most intense part of your **Change**.

### Step 2. Engage the energy . . .

• **Olive** is the Bach flower remedy for exhaustion.

• For every hour you work, take a 60-second break. Breathe deeply; stand up and stretch; change your view; drink some herbal infusion.

★ List ten good things about fatigue, laziness, lethargy, and procrastination. I've found laziness to be my best guide to efficiency; lethargy has stopped me from taking foolish risks; and procrastination helps me find more efficient ways to proceed. Love and honor your fatigue for helping you conserve energy and giving you time to find creative *new     ways     to     do     the     same     old     things.*

### Step 3. Nourish and tonify

• **Seaweeds** of all kinds help restore energy by nourishing nervous, immune, and hormonal systems. Make it a habit to eat some every day.

★ When you feel bone-tired, get grounded energy with **ginseng, black cohosh, yellow dock,** or **dandelion** roots. Use 5-10 drops of the tincture of any *one* of these with each meal for several weeks.

• **Stir** up your wise blood so it doesn't just sit there making you feel exhausted. Stand up, feet shoulder-width, knees relaxed. Swing the arms toward the opposite side. Let the shoulders and hips move as you twist the upper body. Let the arms move freely. After a minute or two, stop, and rock the tail bone and pelvis forward and back, forward and back for at least a minute. Repeat several times a day.

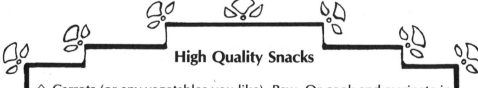

## High Quality Snacks

◇ Carrots (or any vegetables you like). Raw. Or cook and marinate in "Old Sour Puss Mineral Mix" (see page 192) and some olive oil.

◇ Fresh or dried unsulfured fruits, applesauce.

◇ Seaweeds such as toasted dulse or crunchy kelp. Toast dulse in a cast-iron frying pan with a little oil. Yum.

◇ Whole grain pretzels, crackers, chips, rice cakes.

◇ Herbal infusions.

◇ Low-fat cheese, yogurt, almonds.

★ **Green** is the color of plant energy. The plants with the deepest green give you the most energy. A daily cup of **nettle** infusion increases energy without wiring your nerves.

• An evening cup of **oatstraw** infusion builds deep energy for the next day, especially when you have been riding an emotional roller coaster.

• **Eat more.** When you're too tired to eat, you get more tired. (If this sounds like an old wives' tale, remember that old wives were the wise women. But, actually, it's the latest scientific thinking.) In addition to at least one really good meal a day, eat high quality snacks hourly.

*Step 4. Stimulate/Sedate . . .*

★ Though it seems contrary, **St. Joan's wort** (*Hypericum*) tincture relaxes the nerves yet increases energy. Take 25-30 drops several times a day, including before bed, and you'll sleep better, ache less, and wake up with more energy and a brighter outlook on life.

• Warming herbs such as **cayenne, ginger,** and **cinnamon** increase energy (but may increase hot flashes, too). Make a tea with 1 cup/250 ml boiling water and ½-1 teaspoonful (1-2 grams) of the powder of any one of these.

• Some menopausal women report greater fatigue on days when they've eaten frozen food, raw food, or animal products (especially meat). Tradional Chinese Medicine says eating chilled foods, especially cold or iced drinks, contributes to fatigue by using your internal energy to warm the food, and suggests using a stove instead of your stomach.

• **Wheat grass** juice, **green barley** powder, **spirulina,** and **blue green algae** are stimulating and energizing. Use small amounts for best long-term results.

*Step 5a. Use supplements . . .*

• **Vitamin E**, up to 1,300 IU daily, and **vitamin B** complex, up to 50 mg daily, are suggested to remedy fatigue.

• Low levels of **potassium, iron,** and **iodine** contribute to fatigue. Supplemental levels as high as 6000 mg potassium, 100 mg iron, and 100 micrograms iodine have been recommended.

*Step 5b. Use drugs . . .*

• "Energy-producing" foods/drugs such as coffee and candy are not recommended for menopausal women.

• Pharmaceutical drugs that increase energy are not recommended, either.

# Headaches/Migraine

*"Oh, how densely packed your head is, my sweet," sighs Grandmother Growth. "I'm afraid there's no room for new growth. If you could empty your mind, leave off worrying and planning for a while, and give in to chaos and its random pleasures, just for a short time, I think you'd feel less pressure and your head would hurt less. The energy of your womb now circulates inside you and throbs in your head. Sit quietly; breathe out through the top of your head and imagine the breath falling gently down to earth. Rest your forehead against the earth. Place this cool stone on your third eye. Your Crone's Crowning comes closer. This is the work of your body; let your mind rest."*

### Step 0. Do nothing . . .

★ Follow your natural instinct when pained by headache: lie in total silence, in complete darkness, and sleep, if possible, until the headache is gone.

★ Like fatigue, a headache, especially a migraine, is a way to get some **time alone**. Is finding time for yourself usually a headache?

### Step 1. Collect information . . .

Menopause often brings relief to the woman who has had migraine headaches since adolescence. Other women experience headaches for the first time during menopause, usually the result of fatigue, stress, rapidly changing hormone levels racing through the liver, and rushes of kundalini moving into the crown area.

Menopausal headaches may also be triggered by sudden (and usually short-lived) allergies to certain foods.

Headaches and migraines are a common side effect of ERT/HRT.

### Step 2. Engage the energy . . .

• Rub a drop of essential oil of **lavender** or **chamomile** briskly between your hands. When your palms are warm and tingly, place them on the part of your head that aches. (It's also wonderful to have someone do this for you.)

• If it's tolerable for someone to hold your head, try this: Sit in a chair or lie down. Lean your head back into your friend's hands and allow them to support your head in their palms (fingers pointing down, thumbs above ears) for up to five minutes. Breathe fully.

★ A study showed that women who looked at **blinking red lights** relieved their migraines within an hour 72 percent of the time, even when they rated the intensity of the headache extreme or severe. Wear goggles that restrict side vision for maximum effect.

★ Women with chronic migraines often benefit greatly from the help of a skilled feminist therapist.

### Step 3. Nourish and tonify . . .

★ A tea, infusion, or tincture of **garden sage** leaves offers immediate relief from a headache and helps prevent future ones.

★ **Black cohosh** root tincture or a vinegar of fresh **willow leaves** will ease a headache with pain-killing methyl salicylate. Ten drops of the tincture or one teaspoon/15 ml of the vinegar is equivalent to two aspirin.

★ **Vervain** (*Verbena officinalis*) was a sacred herb in the ancient matriarchies. Menopausal women use the tincture of fresh vervain flowers, 20-40 drops in water, before bed and as needed, to strengthen the nerves, relieve insomnia, dispel depression, treat nervous exhaustion, and moderate headaches, including migraines. (Vervain was a favored plant for the Maiden's altar and the moon lodge, where she was used to promote the onset of the menstrual flow, ease cramps, reduce flooding, and quicken desire.)

• **Lady's mantle**, another ancient sacred plant, has many magical attributes, including an ability to aid women who are taking on or leaving the role of mother. What a wonderful friend for an emerging crone! Try 10-25 drops of the tincture of the fresh herb several times a day to relieve headaches.

• The beautiful spring **primrose** (*Primula veris*) offers relief from menopausal headaches if taken regularly. The golden carpet of Schlesselblume on Bavarian pastures and roadsides is one of my favorite memories of Germany. If you don't visit or live in Bavaria, you can grow and gather the blossoms of *Primula officinalis* instead; they're also a good source of pain-killing salicyn. Make a tea of the dried flowers and drink several cups a day for some months. CAUTION: Sip your first cup mindfully and slowly, as some folks are allergic to primrose. NOTE: The roots of most primroses contain oil-soluble estrogenic factors and cell-softening saponins, suggesting use as an ointment for tender, dry vaginal tissue.

★ Chronic headaches as well as sudden headaches can be triggered by a variety of foods, alone or in combinations, particularly: citrus fruit; yogurt; aged cheese; miso; liver; cured meats such as ham; red wine; aspartame; MSG; chocolate; and the nightshade family (tomatoes, potatoes, eggplant, peppers, tobacco). It may take 24-36 hours before the onset of the headache.

### Step 4. Sedate/Stimulate . . .

• Sedate the pain of a headache with **skullcap** tincture, 3-5 drops, and **St. Joan's wort** tincture, 25-30 drops. You can take both herbs together as frequently as needed, up to half a dozen times a day. For migraine sufferers: take as soon as the aura begins, before there is pain, and repeat every ten minutes for 3-6 doses.

• Herbs that are anti-inflammatory and hormone-rich, such as **wild yam**, are the boon companions of menopausal women with headaches. Wild yam root is taken tinctured, 10-30 drops up to 6 times a day, or infused, 1-2 teacupsful a day. Use the lower dose to help relieve chronic headaches. In acute situations, use the higher dose. In addition to preventing and easing headaches, wild yam soothes the urinary tract, eases nausea, and helps balance hormones.

• **Soak your feet** in hot water, especially if scented with a few drops of **rosemary oil**. Rub both small toes around the nail. This stimulates blood flow in the extremities and relieves congestion in your head.

• Migraines are most frequent between 6 AM and noon. Taking herbal medicines before bed and on awakening will insure maximum effect.

• Soak a handful of fresh **lemon balm** (*Melissa*) leaves in a glass of wine for an hour or more (or, less effective, make a tea of dried leaves). Drink to banish simple headaches. Substitute catnip (*Nepeta cataria*) if you want sleep along with your headache cure.

• **Feverfew** (*Chrysanthemum parthenium*) has been much publicized as a remedy for migraine. It is most effective when a sprig of the fresh plant is eaten daily as a preventative measure. For acute headache, try eating 2-4 fresh leaves. If this irritates your mouth, make tea from dried leaves. Drink up to a cup a day.

### Step 5a. Use supplements . . .

• Supplemental **magnesium** and **vitamin B$_6$** may help reduce headaches.

### Step 5b. Use drugs . . .

• Aspirin and other painkillers are many women's first thought as a remedy for headache. But habitual use may actually increase the duration and frequency of headaches.

• Are you taking ERT/HRT? Ease off and see if your headaches ease up.

### Step 6. Break and enter . . .

• Some women say that their headaches are so bad they want to blow their brains out. Perhaps menopausal headaches, like sleeplessness, are part of the physical "mind-altering" process of becoming a crone.

# Heart Palpitations

*"All of your energies are changing, dear one," affirms Grandmother Growth. "Your heart is changing. It is expanding into the broad heart of the self-initiated Crone, who honors excitement and thrills, as well as calm and subtlety. This part of the journey may make your heart pound.*

*"Do your palpitations bring up thrilling memories and quivering fears, which are also your secret desires?*

*"Listen to your heart. Let the energy of your uterus spiral strongly into your heart. Nourish your heart, young Crone, so she can beat strongly for many more years and carry you into very old age."*

**Step 1. Collect information . . .**

Heart palpitations (a pounding, racing pulse of up to 200 beats a minute) may accompany flashes during the menopausal years. Palpitations are not indicative of heart disease. Their genesis during menopause is unclear. They may be caused by electrolyte imbalances from fluid loss if you sweat frequently and heavily. They may also be triggered by strenuous exercise and strong emotions.

It is not surprising that menopausal **Change** affects the heart as well as the uterus, for they are very similiar organs: both are smooth muscle tissue and they both produce some hormones. The uterus is the strongest muscle in a woman's body; the heart is the strongest muscle in a man's body.

Herbs that treat the uterus treat the heart as well. The healing color for the uterus is red; for the heart, green. Plants that strengthen heart/uterus are often green/red: for instance, hawthorn, rose, strawberry, and raspberry, and motherwort.

NOTE: If you have a minor heart valve prolapse (10 percent of the population does), it may suddenly be noticeable at menopause, when the prolapse allows palpitations. Seek expert help if your palpitations leave you extremely breathless, very dizzy, or in great pain.

**Step 2. Engage the energy . . .**

★ **Rose** flower essence calms and steadies the heart.

★ Close your eyes. Put one hand on your heart, the other on your belly or solar plexus. Breathe slowly for 2-5 minutes or until your heart beat is even and quiet.

**Step 3. Nourish and tonify . . .**

★ **Hawthorn** (*Crataegus*) is one of the slowest-acting but most reliable heart tonics known. (It also remedies insomnia.) Hawthorn shrubs and trees are found the world over, providing plenty of fresh and dried berries for tinctures. Try 25-40 drops up to four times a day and don't expect results for over a month.

★ Fluid loss from hot flashes and night sweats can causes palpitations. Drink lots of water; better yet, mineral-rich herbal infusions; best, fresh organic **grape juice** or grapes. Keep some by your bed to drink when you wake in the night and first thing in the morning.

★ **Motherwort** tincture, 10-20 drops with meals and before bed, tones the heart and helps prevent palpitations. Or try 25-50 drops for immediate relief when your heart is pounding crazily.

*"My mother is astonished, and relieved, that motherwort so dependably stops her irregular, wild heart beats, a frightening experience for her. And there it is, growing right outside her bedroom window, planted by the Great Creator."*

★ **Black haw** (*Viburnum*) root bark exerts an antispasmodic effect on the heart and uterus and supplies phytosterols as well. It's all a menopausal woman with a racing heart could want. Sip the infusion frequently or try 25 drops of tincture. NOTE: Although black haw contains some blood-thinning coumarins, experience has shown it unlikely to promote flooding during menopause (or while giving birth).

### Step 4. Sedate/Stimulate . . .

★ **Valerian** root tea by the mouthful, or tincture by the dropperful, promptly slows and eases racing hearts.

• **Ginger** root tea, hot or cold, warms, soothes, and calms the heart. It may, however, increase sweating and flooding.

• A piece of real **licorice** (the root, not the candy) to chew on when your heart starts to race will exert an antispasmodic effect and enrich your estrogen levels, too. CAUTION: Prolonged use may elevate blood pressure, increase fluid retention, and upset bowels.

• Habits such as heavy smoking, large intake of caffeine, or regular use of alcohol increase the severity and incidence of palpitations during the menopausal years.

### Step 5a. Use supplements . . .

★ **Vitamin E** (200-1200 IU daily) is frequently recommended as a remedy for menopausal palpitations. Regular internal use of vitamin E keeps skin pliable and delays wrinkles, too. (Caution: page 62.)

★ **Magnesium**, especially the more absorbable, less laxative types (like magnesium glyconate) are very relaxing to the chest, heart, and lungs. Daily use of 500 mg, taken between meals, helps prevent palpitations and deepens sleep.

*Step 5b. Use drugs . . .*

• Heart palpitations may be caused by antihistamines such as Benadryl, Nyquil, Dimetapp.

• In the rare cases when there is an underlying physical reason for palpitations, drugs may be helpful. Seek skilled help.

*Step 6. Break and enter . . .*

• Invasive diagnostic tests are not recommended for the woman who experiences menopausal palpitations.

# Preventing Breast Cancer

The menopausal years begin the peak years for breast cancer. Three-quarters of all breast cancers occur in women over 50. The death rate from breast cancer is the same now as it was 50 years ago.

It is beyond the scope of this book to deal adequately with remedies for breast cancers. (There are many kinds of breast cancer.) Please refer to the fourth book in this series, *Wise Woman Ways for Women Who Love Their Breasts & Uterus and Don't Want to Lose Them,* for a full discussion of breast cancer and remedies.

To reduce the risk of developing breast cancer:

☞ **Reduce dietary fat.**

No large-scale studies have shown conclusively that breast cancer is caused by a high-fat diet, but numerous studies have shown that a low-fat diet is linked with lower incidence of breast cancer. Note that cancer-promoting hormone residues from growth hormones added to animal food are concentrated in the animals' fat cells. The best way to cut down on fat: eliminate or reduce meat and high-fat cheeses in your diet, unless from organic sources, and even then, use sparingly.

☞ **Don't take supplemental hormones.**

There is little question about the connection between ERT and increased rates of breast cancer. It is only a matter of how great an increase. There are no figures that all authorities in the field agree on.

There is general consensus, however, that the longer the estrogen therapy, the greater the cancer risk.

The highest figures I found showed women who take ERT for 2-5 years have 38 percent more breast cancer than those who don't; 5-9 years of ERT increased breast cancers by 55 percent; and 10 years of ERT produced a 70 percent increase. The lowest figures I found showed little or no increase in breast cancer for women using ERT for fewer than 5 years, and a 30-35 percent increase in women using it for more than 5 years. (To be effective in controlling osteoporosis, ERT must be taken for at least 15 years, or from the last menses until roughly the age of seventy. Some doctors advise taking ERT for the rest of your life.)

Preliminary figures also show increased incidence of breast cancer in women taking HRT.

☞ **Don't have mammograms; do examine your breasts regularly.**

A mammogram may help *find* cancer (by revealing suspicious masses in the breasts that are too small to feel) but it cannot *prevent* it. Repeated mammograms may even cause breast cancers. A mammogram, with 250-300 millirads of radiation per dose, is one of the three highest-dose X-ray procedures currently done. (For comparison, an upper GI series, with swallowed barium, is 150-400 millirads; a lower GI series, with barium enema, is 90-250.) It is a given that damage from radiation includes cancerous changes in cells. *Of all the body tissues, breast cells are among those most easily damaged by radiation.*

Breast self-examination is much less expensive than a mammogram, as reliable in detecting cancer if done consistently and thoroughly, and has no potential for causing cancer. Professional help in breast self-exam, initially and as a regular back-up, improves your chances of detecting cancers.

☞ **Eat tofu.**

Chinese women have half the breast cancers that American women do. One reason seems to be their very low-fat diets; another appears to be regular consumption of tofu and other soy products. Researchers note that high dietary intake of foods rich in phytosterols/phyto-estrogens (such as tofu and yams) seems to suppress the body's production of the estrogens that feed hormone-dependent cancers.

# References & Resources
## Chapter 2: This Is Menopause!

"A Book About Menopause," Montreal Health Press, 1988

"Botanical Applications of Gynecological Conditions," Cascade A. Geller, Tape G15-400, $10 postpaid, Tree Farm Communications, 23703 NE 4th Street, Redmond, WA 98053. (They also have Susun Weed tapes.)

"Botanical Treatment of Chronic Gynecological Conditions, Including Symptoms of Menopause," Silena Heron, 1989 (unpublished paper).

"Can Drugs Treat Menopause?," Jane Brody in *The New York Times*, May 19, 1992 (Front page, Science Times.)

"A Change of Thought on Change of Life," Carol Saline, Philadelphia Magazine, January 1992

"The Estrogen Question," Consumer Reports, September 1991

"Estrogen Therapy: Rx for Nearly All Women," Johns Hopkins Medical Letter/Health After 50, March 1992

"The Gift of Menopause," Anon., 1981

"Good News About Menopause," C. Raymond, in American Health, Nov., 1988

"Homeopathic Medicine For Women," T. Smith, MD, Healing Arts, 1989

Hot Flash, Vol. 1, #1: Holistic Approaches; Vol. 6, #4: Menopause.

"Medical SelfCare Book of Women's Health," Bobbie Hassilbring, Sadja Greenwood, MD, & M. Castleman, Doubleday, 1987 • Scant on alternative answers, heavy on ERT.

"Menopause," Paula Weideger et al., Health Right, 1975

"Menopause: If It Isn't Broken, Don't Fix It," Linda Showler, letter to Townsend Letter for Doctors, printed in the May, 1990 issue.

"Menopause Changed My Life," Diana Siegal, in Sojourner, March 1991

"Menopause: The Closure of Menstrual Life," Ann Voda & Mona Eliasson, from "Lifting the Curse of Menstruation," Haworth, 1983

"Menopause: A Dance Between Delight and Regret," Donaleen Saul, in ANIMA, Vol. 18, #1, Fall 1991

"Menopause: Dreadful Affliction or Glorious Experience," Paavo Airola, in Let's Live, July 1976

"Menopause: A Journey Homeward," Connie Batten, Woman of Power #14, 1989

"Menopause, Naturally," Sadja Greenwood, Volcano Press, 1984 • Easy, helpful, but no index and lots of space devoted to ERT.

"Menopause Naturally," Judyth Reichenberg-Ullman, Natural Health Magazine, March 1992

"Menopause, A Positive Approach," Rosetta Reitz, Penguin, 1979

"The Menopause Rag," Phyllis Orrick in *New York Press*, Vol. 5, #4, June 1992.
"Menopause, A SelfCare Manual," Judy Costlow, Maria Christina Lopez, Mara Taub, Santa Fe Health Education Project, 1991
"The Menopause Self-Help Book," Susan Lark, MD, Celestial Arts, 1990
"Menopause without Medicine," Linda Ojeda, Hunter House, 1989
"Natural Healing in Gynecology," Rina Nissim, Pandora, 1986
"Natural Health Remedies," Pela Sander, in "Women of the 14th Moon," cited below.
"New Directions in Menopause," HealthFacts, Vol. XIV, #126, Nov. 1989
"Second Spring: A Guide To Healthy Menopause through Traditional Chinese Medicine," Honora Lee Wolfs, Blue Poppy, 1990
"Silent Passage: Menopause," Gail Sheehy, Random House, 1992 • See excellent critique in "The Menopause Rag."
"Take This Book to the Gynecologist with You: A Consumer's Guide to Women's Health," Gale Maleskey, Addison-Wesley, 1991
"For Women of All Ages," SH Cherry, MD, Macmillan, 1979
"Women's Health Alert," SM Wolfe, MD, Addison Wesley, 1991
"Women of the 14th Moon: Writing on Menopause," ed. Dena Taylor & Amber Sumrall, Crossing, 1991 • Highly recommended.
"Women on Menopause," Anne Dickson & Nikki Henriques, Healing Arts, 1988

# Herbal Allies for Women in the Midst of Menopause

Here, without further ado, are seven wonderful herbal allies that I and other practitioners find exceptionally useful for women in the midst of **Change:** black cohosh, chaste tree, liferoot, sage, motherwort, ginseng, and Dang Gui.

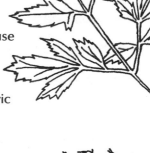

## Black Cohosh
*Cimicifuga racemosa*
Schwarze Sclangenwurzel, Cimicifuga
(Chinese herbalists use Sheng Ma: *C. foetida, C. dahurica*, and others.)

This stately and striking plant of the hardwood forest has long been used by Native Americans, who consider it a powerful plant ally for menopausal women. Science agrees. A study done in Germany in 1988 showed regular use of black cohosh tincture to be as effective as ERT in mitigating common menopausal problems such as hot flashes, headaches, joint pain, water retention, and fatigue.

Use black cohosh during your menopausal years to:

• *Reduce intensity and frequency of hot flashes*
• *Support and ease your menopausal metamorphosis*
Black cohosh supplies estrogenic sterols, gly-cosides, and an amazing array of micronutrients that help you produce and use all kinds of hormones. Use of 10-15 drops once or twice a day for several months significantly reduces LH but not FSH.

• *Help counteract menopausal prolapses*
American and European herbalists say regular use of black cohosh tonifies and strengthens pelvic muscles, preventing and correcting uterine and bladder prolapses. Oriental herbalists also hold it in high regard for treatment of pelvic prolapse.

• *Improve digestion*
Black cohosh increases your digestive juices. Use 3-5 drops with meals.

- *Relieve menstrual pain and menstrual irregularity*
- *Relieve headaches*
- *Relieve menopausal arthritis and rheumatism*

Antispasmodic factors and aspirin-like salicylates that dilate the blood vessels (constricted blood vessels are a common reason for headaches) as well as constituents that slightly depress the central nervous system make black cohosh a superb reliever of pain. Use 15-25 drops as needed.

- *Relieve angina pain*

Cardiotonic black cohosh lowers the blood pressure, improves circulation, causes dilation of the blood vessels, and thins the blood. For acute use, try 25-30 drops as needed. To tonify, use 10 drops daily.

- *Increase energy, calm the nerves, ease hysteria, bring sleep*

Long praised as a potent remedy for hysterical women, black cohosh is also an energy tonic: it invigorates the chi and helps balance the nerves. Try 5-10 drops a day as a long- term tonic; 25 drops as a sedative.

- *Alleviate water retention and breast tenderness*
- *Treat incontinence*

By nourishing the kidneys and adrenals, black cohosh eases fluid buildup. And by stopping spasms in the urinary system, black cohosh successfully treats incontinence.

Pungent, bittersweet, fall-dug black cohosh roots are banned from the supper table and relegated to the apothecary, where they are used in teas and tinctures.

**Dosage:** **Infusion of dried root, up to a teacup a day, by the spoonful.**
    **Tincture of the fresh rhizome/roots, 10-60 drops, daily.**

DO NOT USE black cohosh if you have menstrual flooding or suspect you may be pregnant. The irritating effects (headache, dizziness, visual disturbance, nausea) of black cohosh and other members of the buttercup family are more common and more troublesome in preparations made from dried, powdered roots.

# Vitex or Chaste Tree
## *Vitex agnus-castii*
(Chinese herbalists use Man Jing Zi: *Vitex rotundifolia* or *V. trifolia.*)

Recommended for mid-life women since antiquity, vitex is an especially important ally for today's woman whether she achieves menopause naturally or through surgery, radiation, or drugs.

It is most legendary as an anti-aphrodisiac to men, however, hence the names "chaste tree" and "monk's pepper." Does it affect women this way? The verdict isn't in and the evidence is mixed. Vitex may actually be an aphrodisiac to the female system.

Daily use of vitex berry tincture has been shown to enhance some hormones: progesterone, leutinizing hormone, and luteotropic hormone, but to inhibit others: follicle stimulating hormone and prolactin. (It also increases production of the brain chemical dopamine.) Whether it makes him droop or you horny, vitex does have a powerful effect on the endocrine glands.

But not a fast effect. Vitex contains flavonoids, glycosides, and micronutrients, but lacks phytosterols, making it a slow-acting tonic. Results become evident only after two or three months of daily use; permanent improvement requires about a year's commitment.

It's worth your patience. Use vitex during your menopausal years to:

• *Reduce and eliminate severe hot flashes and dizziness*
Vitex is especially useful for the woman who flashes due to high levels of estrogen and FSH.

• *Reduce and eliminate endometriosis and uterine fibroids*
• *Relieve chronic menstrual cramps*
Regular use of vitex berry tincture has a pronounced anti-inflammatory effect on the endometrium. Numerous herbalists in America and England report slow but steady remission of fibroids in women using vitex regularly for 1-2 years.

• *Eliminate flooding, spotting, and irregular cycles*
Vitex is an incredible nourisher to the pituitary gland, which controls and coordinates the menstrual cycle. When flooding and spotting are from a corpus luteum deficiency, ally with vitex.

• *Redirect hysteria into focused action and emotional calm*
Hysteria (literally: "wild womb energy") can be usable energy. Try vitex for slow, steady regrounding; motherwort for acute care.

• *Clear skin problems*
Acne related to hormonal changes often disappears after even a few weeks of regular vitex consumption. Allergic skin disturbances often clear with regular use, too.

• *Relieve hormone-related constipation and digestive distresses*
As in pregnancy, the muscular movements of the digestive tract slow during menopause. Vitex cures and prevents this sluggishness.

• *Lessen tenderness and lumps in the breasts*
• *Relieve water retention and tissue distension (edema and bloat)*
• *Eliminate headaches, migraines, and depression*
Virtually all the typical PMS symptoms are relieved, and ultimately cured, with regular use of vitex for six to thirteen months. To avoid relapse continue for three to six months after all symptoms are gone.

• *Protect against reproductive cancers (may help cure)*
• *Reestablish menstruation that has stopped prematurely*
• *Protect against osteoporosis*
• *Treat dry vaginal tissues*
Vitex gently lowers estrogen levels (protecting reproductive tissues from cancers), and increases progesterone levels (keeping bones and vaginal walls strong).

Though not native to North America, vitex bushes are easily grown here. Use the fresh or dried berries infused in water or alcohol (tinctured). If vitex is your menopausal ally and it doesn't grow near you, buy a whole pound of the berries; you'll use them.
**Dosage: 20 drops tincture 1-2 times daily.**
**3 capsules freshly powdered berries daily.**
**1 cup/250ml tea of freshly powdered berries daily.**
In use for over 2000 years in Northern Africa, vitex has a reputation for being free of side effects.

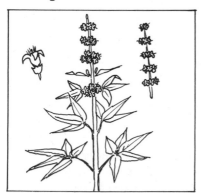

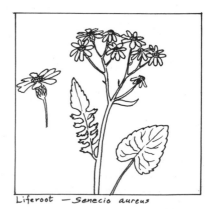

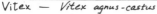
Vitex — *Vitex agnus-castus*      Liferoot —*Senecio aureus*

# Liferoot
*Senecio aureus*
# Groundsel
*Senecio vulgaris*
Gemeines Kreuzkraut, Séneçon Commun
# Jacob's Groundsel
*Senecio jacobaea*
Jacobskraut, Séneçon Jacobée

The *Senecios* have a bad reputation for poisoning livestock, but a great reputation for helping women during menopause, birth, and menstrual distress.

These glycoside-rich "troublesome perennial weeds" are good sources of phytosterols. Many authors warn against their use, but I have seen nothing but favorable results with small doses of the blossom tincture. Liferoot and groundsel are classic tonics, having far greater effect over a long time than as quick-acting remedies. Use daily for two weeks out of each month for at least two months before expecting to see results.

Use any one of the *Senecios* during the menopausal years to:

• *Completely eliminate severe menstrual pain, nausea, debility*
Liferoot is an ally without peer for women incapacitated by chronic severe menstrual distress. For best effect, take 5-8 drops daily for two weeks before your bleeding begins.

• *Moderate hot flashes*
• *Tonify the uterine muscle*
• *Regulate the menstrual cycle, slow flooding, cure anemia*
Powerful plant hormones and an ability to increase circulating iron are the gifts of liferoot. *Senecio* is considered safe to use even if you flood.

• *Soothe the nerves, moderate emotional swings*
• *Relieve PMS symptoms, especially breast tenderness*
• *Reduce gravel and other urinary tract problems*
• *Increase libido*
*Senecios* choose to grow where they can collect a wide spectrum of trace elements and micronutrients, which slowly accumulate in your body as you consume them, balancing and nourishing the nerves, endocrine system (including adrenals), and kidneys. Once all of these are in top shape, the libido kicks in. I've seen it happen many times. Don't discount this effect or you may be in for a surprise.

Out of respect for the alkaloids concentrated in the roots, I use only the flowering tops and leaves of liferoot. The lively yellow flowers turn into dandelion-like fluff balls and blow away if dried, so I tincture them in vodka when they bloom in the spring.

**Dosage:** Tincture of fresh flowers, 5-15 drops per day. Best taken during luteal phase only.

CAUTION: *Senecio* can cause temporary (but distressing) changes in your menstrual and premenstrual patterns during the first few months of use.

Barbara didn't have hot flashes at menopause, she had cold sweats. "First I'd be cold, then hollow in my gut, and I'd think I was going to wet my pants I had to pee so bad. Then my heart would pound and I'd be wet from scalp to toe, and really chilled. I'd have to bring changes of clothes with me wherever I went, I'd get so wet so unexpectedly. If I was stressed, I'd get very dizzy, too." She read about Ginseng, bought some whole roots and chewed them "as much as I could for the past three moon cycles." She even cooked them for hours in her soups. "And I just realized I haven't had a chilling sweat in over a week."

Alex had taken estrogen for three years to control her severe hot flashes, and she was ready to try something else. Since she'd always gotten chilled after her flashes, had been anemic off and on, and really liked celery and cilantro, she decided to ally with Dang Gui. "For the first few weeks, I took a little Dang Gui with my whole dose of ERT. Then I gradually withdrew from the estrogen by cutting my pills to smaller and smaller sizes and eating more Dang Gui."

A year later, Alex is still free of sweats, chills, and flashes, and is considering cutting out the Dang Gui as well.

# Garden Sage
### *Salvia officinalis*
Salbei, Sauge officinale, Shu Wei T'sao

DO NOT USE sagebrush/desert sage (*Artemisia tridentata*).

*"Where sage doth grow well and vigorous, therein rules a strong woman."*                                    *–Old wives' saying*

The ancients called sage sacred. *Salvia* means the savior. Since ancient times, sage has dried breast milk and stopped menopausal sweating, eased the minds and wombs and bellies of women everywhere. There is no other herb so effective at drying up the flowing springs of perspiration that gush with some women's hot flashes. But that's not all.

Use garden sage during the menopausal years to:

• *Eliminate night sweats, cold sweats, and hot flash sweats*
The effect is generally noticeable within two hours and can continue for a day or more from a single dose. In TCM, Traditional Chinese Medicine (a Wise Woman tradition), sweat is regarded as a precious pure fluid of life and a cooling substance.

• *Regulate hormonal* **Change**
Sage's estrogenic effects have long been noted; our oldest foremothers used it to increase fertility. Sage contains flavonoids and phytosterols.

• *Ease irritated nerves, banish depression*
Mineral-consolidating sage is rich in mellow calcium, calming magnesium, peppy potassium, sexy zinc, and anti-stress thiamine.

• *Relieve dizziness, trembling, and emotional swings*
Sweating doesn't remove toxins from the body, but it does remove minerals. When you sweat profusely, the mineral loss can cause dizziness, trembling, emotional swings, and even joint pain. Sage not only stops sweating and the resulting mineral loss, its rich mineral reserves help you make up for previous depletion.

• *Eliminate headaches*
Sage contains headache-easing saponins, which keep the blood flowing freely; carotenes, which nourish the liver (in TCM, headaches are related to liver weakness); and essential fatty acids, which keep the blood vessels flexible.

• *Strengthen the liver, aid digestion, decrease excess gas*
Like its sister mints — peppermint, rosemary, thyme, spearmint and savory — sage is rich in essential oils that help the stomach and liver produce more digestive enzymes and acids, thus easing indigestion, nausea, and gas.

• *Relieve menstrual cramps and flooding*
Sage's antispasmodic oils and sweat-stopping tannins exert their influence all the way to the uterus, giving you prompt relief from pain and excess bleeding.

• *Reduce bladder infections*
Sage contains highly disinfectant oils that concentrate in the urine, discouraging bacterial growth.

• *Prevent joint aches, improve circulation*
Sage's essential fatty acids and minerals are boons to those suffering from aching joints. When you receive optimum minerals from herbs, mineral deposits at your joints are more likely to dissolve into the blood. Sage's saponins also grease your joints and ease inflammation.

• *Gain mental clarity, a strong memory, and a calm "craziness"*
One who is wise is a sage. To burn sage is to clear the air. In legend, to rub a person with sage kept them safely in a transformed state. The Crone is so sane she is sometimes considered mentally odd. Breathe in the deep scent of sage and welcome the crazy old crone you are becoming.

• *Slow the aging process*
Sage lives up to its seemingly absurd claim of bestowing extra decades of life on its users: it is antiseptic to most bacteria inside (and on) your body, filled with antioxidants that retard wrinkles and grey hair and help prevent cancer, blessed with heart-healthy oils, abundant with much-needed minerals, and easy to grow, even in a pot. Why not make a cup of sage tea, right now?

Powerful-tasting sage is a welcome additon to whole grain and vegetable dishes (and, yes, turkey stuffing). Try fresh sage finely chopped and sprinkled on salads, potatoes, carrots, parsnips, beans. Be generous with dried sage in soups; use it as a condiment at the table. Infused, sage makes a dye-like rinse to keep hair dark, an antiseptic rinse for infected gums, and a tasty drink.
**Dosage: 1-2 spoonfuls of dried leaf infusion, 1-8 times daily.**
**15-40 drops of fresh leaf tincture, 1-3 times a week.**
DO NOT USE if you have dry mouth or very dry vaginal tissues. Do not use excessively. The essential oils in sage can accumulate in the kidneys and liver.

# Motherwort
*Leonurus cardiaca*
Herzgespan, Agripaume cardiaque, Yi Mu Cao

"Everyone ought to have a little Mother around the house," Grandmother Edith would frequently say. The Mother she meant is motherwort, a locally common weed and a treasured ally to women stressed by menopausal problems. Grandmother Edith's love affair with motherwort began when her hot flashes knocked her out in the supermarket, continued as it mended her husband's heart, and grew and grew as her five daughters found relief from PMS and menstrual cramps, constipation and the crazies with the help of the little Mother, motherwort.

Use motherwort regularly during the menopausal years to:

• *Lessen the severity, frequency, and duration of hot flashes*
Motherwort regulates and tonifies the functioning of the thyroid, blood vessels, liver, heart, and uterus. For best results use motherwort frequently for 3 months. But don't neglect to try a dropperful (in a splash of water) even after a flash has begun.

• *Relieve faintness with flashes*
Motherwort is traditionally used to relieve shortness of breath and congestion in the respiratory passages. She invigorates the circulation and increases oxygen in the blood. Use the standard dose as soon as you feel faint or dizzy.

• *Ease stressed nerves, relieve anxiety*
Motherwort calms, supports, and strengthens you the way the smell of your mother did when you were very young. Used regularly, motherwort feeds your nerves and your good common sense, relaxing and unclenching any held tension. Motherwort is not sedating, but calming, leaving you ready for action, not flying off the handle or bouncing off the walls. Ask motherwort to be your ally in tough times, in shaky times, in enraging times, in scary times, in depressed times, in grief-filled times. Try 5-10 drops as soon as you feel your nerves starting to fray or just before a stressful event.

• *Relieve insomnia and sleep disturbances*
Use motherwort's high-calcium calming effect when you are awakened by night sweats and have difficulty getting back to sleep. Keep a glass of water and a bottle of motherwort tincture by your bed and take 10-15 drops and a swallow of water as soon as you wake, even if it's three times an hour. Motherwort calms a rapidly beating heart and eliminates the nightmares some women experience with their menopausal Change.

• *Strengthen the heart, reduce palpitations and tachycardia*
Motherwort supplies readily usable minerals, trace elements, and an alkaloid exceptionally tonifying to the heart (and uterus). The German herbal doctor, Weiss, finds motherwort tincture effective treatment for functional heart complaints. The botanical name translates as "lion-hearted." A single dose of motherwort can quickly ease palpitations and tachycardia. Regular use lowers hypertension, and sets you up to be a hale-hearted crone.

• *Eliminate menstrual cramps*
• *Relieve uterine pain*
Motherwort tincture is my favorite remedy for women with uncompli-cated menstrual cramps and a slight to moderate flow (or no flow). I find 5-10 drops usually eases cramps in five to ten minutes. Repeat every ten minutes as needed. Motherwort encourages strong (but not crampy) uterine contractions, which strengthen the uterine muscle. So the more you take motherwort to ease your cramps, the more toned your uterus becomes and the less likely you are to have cramps in the future.

• *Restore thickness and elasticity to vaginal walls*
Motherwort brings blood to the pelvis and thickens all tissues there (bladder, uterus, vagina). Expect noticeable results within the month from 10-15 drop doses taken once or twice a day.

Eva told me that she was having 24-30 powerful hot flashes daily, and that the number and intensity had been consistent for the past two years. She had tried ERT, but it made her feel "miserable, premenstrual." When I visited her, I wasn't sur-prised to find a motherwort "weed" growing in the flower bed beside her front door. It was in full flower; the perfect time to harvest and tincture it.

Six months later, Eva called to tell me she was now having only one or two flashes a day. She'd been taking a dropperful of motherwort tincture 2-4 times a day, and she was involved in the Pathwork (see page 88), which supported her wholeness in very new ways.

"I was always the perfect wife and mother, friend and community member. I never got mad, or even very upset. Last year I had a flash every time someone was rude to me. Mother-wort and the Pathwork have given me permission to be rude back. I thought you said motherwort would make me calm. It didn't; it helped me find my anger."

• *Lift depression*
A dose of motherwort first thing in the morning is far kinder to your system than coffee and helps you ease into the day with a renewed sense of life.

• *Reduce water retention, edema*
Small, frequent doses of motherwort will reduce bloat in a few hours. For longer-term help, use a standard dose once or twice a day for 3-6 weeks.

• *Relieve constipation and extend life*
There is a Japanese saying about the heirs of those who take motherwort: they are grumpy because they must wait so long for their inheritance. But does it really work? A small dose (5-10 drops as needed) does ease gas pain, encourage regular elimination, and improve digestion. That alone would make anyone want to live longer.

Bitter with minerals and alkaloids, motherwort is unwelcome in salads and nasty as an infusion, so it is used as a tincture, vinegar, or syrup. In Oriental herbalism, Yi Mu Cao is cooling, pungent, bitter. *Dosage:* **15-25 drops, tincture of fresh flowering plant, 1-6 times day.**
**1-2 teaspoons/5-10ml vinegar of fresh flowering plant, as desired.**
DO NOT USE if you are experiencing menstrual flooding; motherwort can aggravate this tendency. Do not use daily if you are easily habituated to substances that make you feel really good. Motherwort is so soothing, so calming, that you may begin to lose some of your own standing and lean too heavily on your Mom.

# Ginseng & Dang Gui
## Adaptogenic Roots

*Panax* Ginseng is one of the best known of all herbal medicines. It is more frequently associated with relief from severe menopausal problems, especially hot flashes, than any other herb in Western herbalism.

Dang Gui is the East's most frequently recommended herbal ally for the mid-life woman. Dang Gui is considered by many to be the finest woman's tonic in the world.

Both of these roots specifically support transformation by helping us adapt to **Change**. Unfortunately, they are expensive, difficult or impossible for an amateur to grow, and rare in the wild. Fortunately, they are effective even in very small doses.

Ginseng is yang; it is a chi (energy) tonic. Dang Gui is yin; it is a blood (substance) nourisher. If yang and yin are mistakenly identified as male and female, then we arrive at the common (mistaken) notion that Ginseng is for men and Dang Qui is for women.

Native Americans made no such mistake. Among the Iroquois Nations, Ginseng was well-known as a woman's remedy. The Penobscot Indians also considered it a woman's herb, and advised women wishing to conceive to cook it and eat it.

In fact, both men and women benefit from Ginseng's yang chi tonifying and from Dang Gui's yin blood nourishing, the more so as we age. Blood is the mother of chi; chi is the promoter of blood. Oriental medicine says menopause is the yang (energized) manifestation of yin (wise blood). And we can all benefit from Ginseng and Dang Gui's rich store of minerals, plant hormones, and the B vitamin complex. (Both are sources of $B_{12}$, though there is some question as to whether $B_{12}$ is digestible from plant sources.)

Modern herbalists suggest taking Ginseng for two weeks and then Dang Gui for four weeks, alternating in this fashion for up to two years or until your menopausal transformation is complete. This alternation is highly recommended for women experiencing premature menopause, naturally or through surgery or drugs.

While I generally prefer to use one herb at a time, Chinese herbalists strongly suggest that Dang Gui be taken in combination with other herbs. One of the most ancient and beloved combinations is equal parts of Dang Gui, Rehmannia, Ligusticum, and Peony roots. (See page 194: Dong Quai/Dang Gui Tonic. )

Many herbalists feel that Ginseng should be combined with other roots, too. That's certainly the way the Native Americans used it. (See "Menopausal Root Brew," page 193.)

Sweet, smoky, warm, spicy, exotic, and interesting, the tastes of Ginseng and Dang Gui are intriguing in soups, remarkable in teas, powerful in tinctures, and quite pleasant to chew. The most enjoyable way to purchase Ginseng and Dang Gui is to stroll through Chinatown, stopping at herb stores until you find the roots you want to savor on your journey through menopause.

# Ginseng
## Oriental Ginseng/Ren Shen *Panax ginseng*
## American Ginseng *Panax quinquefolius*
## Tienchi Ginseng *Panax pseudoginseng*
Not "true" ginseng, but used interchangeably:
## Dang Shen *Codonopsis pilosula*
## Siberian Ginseng *Eleutherococcus senticosus*

All varieties of Ginseng are roughly interchangeable in effectiveness. I prefer wild American Ginseng, which is less stimulating, less heating, and perhaps less strongly hormonal than the Ginseng grown in Korea and China.

During the past fifty years, Ginsengs have been the subject of intense scientific scrutiny. For centuries, the indigenous peoples of the lands where the different Ginsengs grow — wild mountainous areas of North America, China, and Russia — have considered them fountains of youth and cure-alls. Science validates their native wisdom: all varieties of Ginseng *are* energizing, rejuvenating (especially to the hormonal system), immuno-protective, and adaptogenic.

Although the benefits of taking Ginseng are cumulative, you'll note improvement in 2–3 weeks if Ginseng is your menopausal ally. The lore of the Catskills (where Ginseng, or 'seng, still grows wild) tells me to chew on a little 'seng spring and fall, and whenever I'm under stress. Since Ginseng is rare in the wild, I use it quite sparingly. The pint of tincture I put up with two large wild roots a few years ago ought to last me the rest of my life.

Wild *Panax* roots, whether American or Chinese, are the most effective of these four Ginsengs. They are the most desired, and most expensive as well. The least effective Ginseng is that bought powdered, in capsules or foil packages. Well-handled commercially grown roots of any Ginseng, dried or tinctured, will offer you maximum effect at the lowest price.

You will neutralize most of Ginseng's effect if you take vitamin C supplements (or eat vitamin C rich foods) within three hours of taking the herb. You will double Ginseng's effects if you take it with 100-200 IU vitamin E or a spoonful of fresh wheat germ oil or flax seed oil.

Take ginseng, especially *Panax*, during the menopausal years to:

• *Reduce the intensity and frequency of hot flashes*
With eleven hormone-like saponins, several phytosterols, and a ready

supply of hormone building blocks such as essential fatty acids, minerals (especially manganese), and glycosides, Ginseng is amply prepared to help ease your menopausal flashes.

• *Improve nervous functions, ease depression and anxiety*
Ginseng is at its best when you are under the most stress. By nourishing the nerves, moderating blood sugar swings, and regulating the hormones, Ginseng helps you use your powerful menopausal emotions instead of being swept away by them.

• *Reduce the effects of stress*
Of all Ginseng's benefits, this is the most demonstrated. When you really can't take a break, and you're burned out, exhausted, numb, clumsy, and feeling dull, make a Ginseng soup, or take the tincture twice a day. Ginseng nourishes and strengthens the adrenal cortex, the pituitary, the thyroid, and the hypothalamus.

• *Stop menstrual flooding, regulate endocrine activity*
The rich supply of plant hormones and micronutrients in Ginseng nourishes your glands and helps you create the estrogen and progesterone you need to continue menstruating regularly, without flooding, until the final period.

• *Improve energy level, reduce fatigue*
Not to be confused with herbal "speeds," which give one a false sense of energy, Ginseng rebuilds your energy and stamina from the inside out by nourishing, regulating, and tonifying virtually all systems. It also lessens fatigue by diminishing night sweats and promoting deeper, more restful sleep.

• *Improve memory, concentration, mental acuity, and clarity*
Ginseng improves mental functioning, especially during stress.

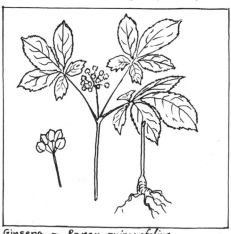

Ginseng — Panax quinquefolius

**• *Normalize blood pressure, reduce cholesterol***
Ginseng's scientifically validated cardiotonic properties nourish your heart and blood vessels, lower elevated blood pressure (without reducing normal blood pressure), increase HDL (high density lipoproteins, the good fats) and reduce LDL (low density lipoproteins, the bad fats).

**• *Reduce the incidence of adult onset diabetes***
Ginseng is particularly valuable for stabilizing blood sugar swings, since it affects the metabolic processes of the liver, and sugar utilization within the muscles.

**• *Eliminate menopausal headaches***
**• *Improve digestion***
For some women, the most distressing menopausal problem is a suddenly sensitive digestive tract. One explanation: the liver is so busy during menopause it can't tend to digestion the way it used to. One remedy: chew on a Ginseng root before or after you eat.

**• *Enhance libido***
Though Ginseng's minerals and hormones may not make you feel like a young doe in heat, you might find yourself having some very "adult" thoughts.

**• *Reduce the aging process, extend the lifespan***
Antioxidants, like rust-resisting paint, slow the oxidation/aging process. Ginseng is full of them.

The taste of Ginseng is sweet, aromatic, and warming, to a greater or lesser degree depending on individual plants and the species. Ginseng roots lend themselves to savory soups, satisfying teas, and robust tinctures, but the classic way to consume Ginseng is to put a piece in your mouth and "just worry it around for an hour or so, until it's all gone."

**Dosage: 5-40 drops of the fresh root tincture 1-3 times daily.**
**4-8 oz/25-50ml dried root infusion or tea daily.**
**Chew a piece of dried root as big as a third of your little finger daily for 6-8 weeks.**

*Note: Dosage varies more with individual plants than among the various species.*

DO NOT USE any Ginseng if you have a fever. DO NOT USE Ginseng, except American, if you feel jittery or have sleep difficulties. Some women report overstimulation with Ginseng: too much energy, a sense of being speeded up, like coffee nerves. There are documented cases of Ginseng causing menstrual-like bleeding long after menopause has culminated. If this happens to you, discontinue use.

# Dang Gui
## *Angelica sinensis*
also spelled: Dong Quai, Tang Kwei, Tang Kuei, Dong Gway

Cherished all over the Orient as a supreme ally for women with reproductive/uterine/hormonal distresses, Dang Gui is now readily available in North America.

Use Dang Gui as a nourishing menopausal ally to:

• *Relieve hot flashes*
A specific for the woman troubled by hot flashes, Dang Gui's sterols and minerals work promptly to modify hot flashes quickly. What's more, these ingredients accumulate in your body, offering more benefit and effectiveness with repeated use. CAUTION: If you feel hot much of the time anyway, Dang Gui is not your ally; ingestion may make you flash all the more.

• *Regulate menses, reduce spotting and flooding*
Dang Gui's intense stores of iron, folic acid, $B_{12}$, and phytosterols will help regulate your cycle and diminish spotting and flooding caused by anemia or lack of hormones. CAUTION: Dang Gui is tricky to use during menopause if you have unpredictable episodes of profuse menstrual bleeding, as it relaxes the uterine muscle and excites contraction (both actions increase the likelihood of flooding). If you flood, you may be able to take Dang Gui except while you are bleeding. Use it daily until you have some premenstrual sign, then stop for a week. If your flooding gets heavier, discontinue use of Dang Gui altogether.

• *Relieve uterine pain*
The sedative and warming qualities of Dang Gui bring warmth and ease to the entire belly, relieving aches or spasms in the uterus or vagina.

• *Revivify thin, dry vaginal tissues*
Dang Gui has long been noted for its ability to move a soothing flow of moisture into the pelvis, hydrating the bowels and easing constipation as well as increasing vaginal secretions, and nourishing and thickening vaginal and bladder walls.

• *Restore a youthful face and complexion*
Dang Gui stirs and heats the blood, and the effect is often immediately obvious in the face, where it gradually plumps out facial wrinkles, and

quickly brings a rosy glow to the cheeks. I once saw a tall thin man drink a cup of Dang Gui broth. As he set the cup down, he flushed from the chest up to his crown (just like a hot flash!) and fainted. We're after a less dramatic effect, however.

• *Reduce headaches, relieve water retention*
Nerve-nourishing, headache-preventing minerals and B vitamins, especially niacin, are plentiful in Dang Gui. As its heating energy moves a flush to the cheeks and an ease to the uterus, it stirs the kidneys to eliminate excess fluid, ending bloat.

• *Eliminate palpitations, decrease heart disease*
Dang Gui is often cited as a remedy for menopausal palpitations. It also reduces high blood pressure and atherosclerosis, and promotes healthy blood circulation. Coumarins in Dang Gui thin the blood much as aspirin does.

• *Ease menopausal insomnia*
Dang Gui improves the quality of your sleep by supplying generous amounts of magnesium, a nerve-mellowing mineral depleted by frequent night sweats.

• *Restore emotional calm*
Dang Gui supplies abundant phytosterols and rare elements such as cobalt to help stabilize emotional upheavals. It also eases nervous irritability caused by hormonal swings and lack of adequate trace minerals.

• *Relieve menopausal rheumatism*
Dang Gui soothes achy joints during (and after) menopause.

• *Tonify the liver*
Free from liver-stressing alkaloids, and rich in liver-nourishing iron, Dang Gui is a grand ally of the liver during the menopausal years.

Dang Gui smells and tastes a little like many of its other family members: celery, lovage, carrot, parsnip, parsley, cilantro, anise, cumin. Dried sliced roots are wonderful to chew on. Garden angelica is related to Dang Gui and is a tolerable substitute, as are wild varieties of angelica, including osha (*Ligusticum porterii*).

**Dosage: 10-40 drops of the fresh root tincture 1-3 times daily.**

**4-8 oz/25-50ml dried root infusion or tea daily.**

**Chew a ⅛-¼ inch (4-6mm) slice of dried root 2-3 times a day.**

DO NOT USE Dang Gui during menstruation if bleeding is heavy. Do not use if you have fibroids. Do not use if you regularly take aspirin or blood-thinning drugs. Do not use if you are bloated. Do not use if you have diarrhea. If you experience extreme breast tenderness or soreness after taking Dang Gui, discontinue use.

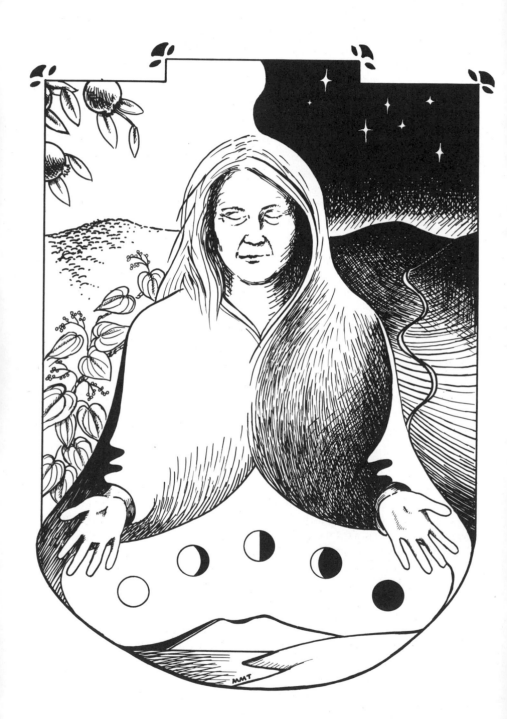

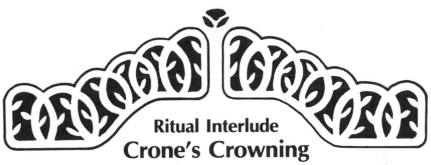

## Ritual Interlude
# Crone's Crowning

The prevalent model of menopause as deficiency disease is hopefully faltering as more and more women find the beauty in their menopause and the power in themselves as Crone, woman of wholeness. Let us not replace that model with one even more injurious to women: that the healthy, well-adjusted woman breezes through menopause with scarcely a problem.

The menopausal years, the climacteric years, constitute an enormous **Change.** And change is a challenge. A challenge each woman will meet in her own unique way. You may feel at times like a stranger in your own body, confused by your own feelings, uncertain and afraid of the **Change** taking place in your own being. You may feel, perhaps with fear, the "you" that you have known for so many years dying, as your last menses become memories.

I know of no herbs, no rituals, no special ways of eating or exercising that will prevent the **Change** of menopause. And, as with puberty, pregnancy, and birth, you may change in ways that are dramatic and difficult to live with. This is not a failing on your part.

In menopause, **Change** is normal; but normal may be difficult, painful. Normal, natural menopause may really hurt, for it is a symbolic death as well as an actual rebirth.

When the pain of labor reaches the ultimate intensity, the child begins at last to come down the birth canal. Slowly or quickly the small body pushes head-first toward its new life. The head at last reaches the vaginal opening; it is crowning.

When the distress of menopause reaches its peak, you begin the push toward your new life. As you reach the outer edge of menopause, you crown yourself Crone.

Your Crone's Crowning ritual marks a change as dramatic as the babe's movement from watery womb dependence to air-breathing independence. You will never again be the same woman you were before you stopped bleeding. As you accept this death, you birth yourself as Crone.

The ritual of Crone's Crowning is the still point before the actual emergence. Umbilicus throbbing, psychically connected yet to the mother you were, you pause before the final push. Your menstrual cycle is finished, forever. Your role as Mother is at an end. Your role as Crone begins with the next breath, the first breath of your new life. To make way for this first breath, the new life, we give death to ourselves as we were.

The following ritual is one way to symbolically encode the death aspect of your menopausal **Change**. I envision you doing this ritual alone or with a group of like-minded women. (This particular ritual is a women's mystery and, as such, does not include men.) I suggest that you do this ritual no sooner than thirteen moons after your very last menses.

*     *     *     *     *

On the night of the new (dark) moon make your way to a place where you feel very safe, very secure. Bring with you pictures, poems, objects, and mementos of your life as a bleeding woman, as Mother (even if you have no children).

Create an altar (sacred space) to woman as mother, she-who-bleeds-and-does-not-die, she-who-creates-from-her-own-blood, she-who-gives-birth-to-all-that-is. Make this altar as beautiful as you can, using lots of flowers and colors. Light three candles, one white (the color of death), one red (the color of life), and one black (the color of fertile possibility). Hum or sing a lullaby while you do this. If you like, place a small statue of the Blessed Virgin Mary or some other symbolic mother on your altar.

Face the altar and breathe toward it. As you inhale, fill yourself with the images, feelings, ideas, thoughts of yourself as Mother. If you have not given birth and feel sad, that is appropriate, as is delight in your choice. If you gave your child away, through adoption or abortion, let the feelings of pain or relief come to the foreground. If you have children, focus on how you feel about your role as their mother.

Call upon the energies of the Mothers of the east, those who sing in new life. Ask them to be present with you. Call upon the energies of the Mothers of the south, those who stoke the fires of new life. Ask them to be present with you. Call upon the energies of the Mothers of the west, those who cry and laugh with life. Ask them to be present with you. Call upon the energies of the Mothers of the north, those who form new life. Ask them to be present with you.

Hold your right hand out in front of you. Look at it carefully as you say: "This is the hand of life. This is the hand of beginnings." Imagine that you hold yourself, as mother, in the palm of your right hand.

Hold your left hand out in front of you. Look at it carefully as you say: "This is the hand of death. This is the hand of endings." Imagine that you hold yourself, as crone, in your left hand.

Looking intently at both of your hands, say, in your own words: "The time for the right hand has come to an end for me. I can no longer give life from my own belly, my own breasts. In the great balance of all that is, I enter now the time for the left hand. I am readying myself to be a giver of death. And though death is a gift that is feared, it is utterly necessary to the continuation of life. As woman it is my privilege to give life and call myself mother. As woman it is my duty to give death and name myself Crone."

Slowly, slowly, bring your hands together, left palm up and above the right hand. "I give death to myself as Mother. I claim my power as Crone." Signify the Mother's death by placing your right hand in a waiting container of mud or clay or brown fingerpaint.

With your left hand, snuff out the red candle. Put the black and white candles to one side, then remove everything else from the altar and place it, with love/relief, grief/joy into a fire or a bucket of water or a trash can. Cry out for the death of your Mother self.

Ask the Crones of the east to come and replace the Mothers of the east. Welcome those who sing the songs of death. Ask the Crones of the south to come and replace the Mothers of the south. Welcome those who stir the cauldron of change and lay the feast for the dead. Ask the Crones of the west to come and replace the Mothers of the west. Welcome those who open the door to death, whose tears shine the way to letting go. Ask the Crones of the north to come and replace the Mothers of the north. Welcome those who silently guard the realm of the dead.

On the bare altar place the two lit candles, black and white, and one hair from your head, a silver one. "I claim myself as Crone. I claim my right to name the end of things." Place upon your head a wreath or crown of your own devising. "I crown myself as Crone. I am she-who-holds-her-wise-blood-inside; I am she-who-walks-with-death."

Thank the Crones, the Mothers, and the energies of the four directions. With your left hand snuff out the black and white candles. In the darkness, hum a lullaby.

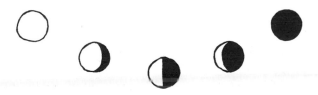

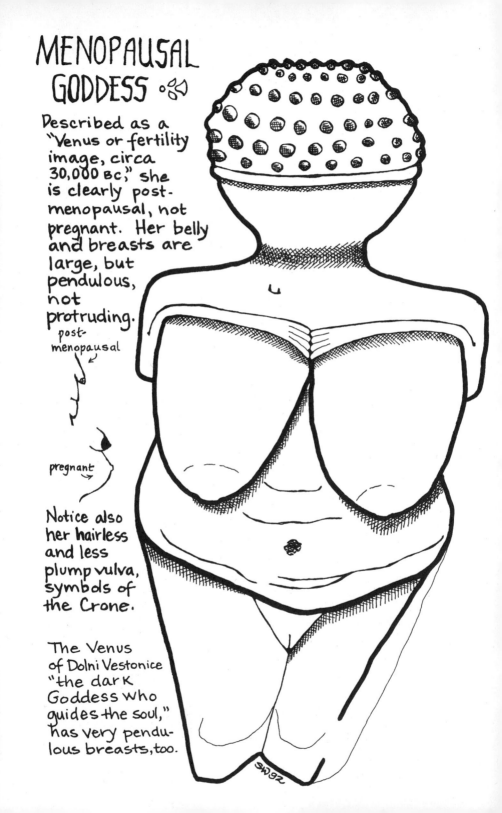

# MENOPAUSAL GODDESS

Described as a "Venus or fertility image, circa 30,000 BC," she is clearly post-menopausal, not pregnant. Her belly and breasts are large, but pendulous, not protruding.

post-menopausal

pregnant

Notice also her hairless and less plump vulva, symbols of the Crone.

The Venus of Dolni Vestonice "the dark Goddess who guides the soul," has very pendulous breasts, too.

SW 92

# Post-Menopause
## She-Who-Holds-Her-Wise-Blood-Inside

*"Soon your voice will merge with my own, dear one," chuckles Grandmother Growth. "We have journeyed long together through this Change, your menopause. And now it is completed. You are crowned Crone. What I have shared with you is imprinted in your cells. Do not be surprised when you look in the mirror and see yourself resembling me.*

*"You are no longer a maiden; but always Maiden, filled with blissful, carefree, poetic energies. You are no longer a mother; but ever Mother, abundant with creative, supportive, life-giving energies. You are now, and all the rest of your days will be, Crone, woman of wholeness, woman of wisdom, she who knows death as well as life, impeccable action as well as spontaneous vitality. And, in time, you will be seen as Grandmother to your community, and Grandmother Growth to new generations of baby Crones.*

*"It is almost time for me to say farewell, granddaughter. But not before I share a few stories with you: stories of flexible bones, and open hearts, and sensual, sexual old age. And not before I urge you to nourish yourself.*

*"There is much for you to do, young Crone. As one of millions of women coming to their Change now, you have a very special place in what some call the 'earth changes.' Yes, granddaughter, by 2013, you and your sister Crones will constitute such a great pool of collective wisdom that you will be able to guide Gaia and her human inhabitants into an amazing new era of global wholeness and personal health."*

You no longer bleed on a monthly basis. Your outer, visible tie to the rhythms of the moon is gone. Now you follow the inner ebb and flow of your own ocean, knowing full well how intimately connected you are to the swells and contractions of the entire universe. You are a post-menopausal woman and again a virgin (she who is owned by no one; not a sexual innocent), freed from any worry about conception, pregnancy, or mothering.

Most of the distresses of your **Change** have faded. Hot flashes are milder, and far less frequent. Creative juices are willing to flow at ordinary hours, allowing a full night's sleep. Your energy levels and emotional levels seem more solid than they've ever been.

Keep taking great care of yourself. In the immediate post-menopausal period, vaginal and bladder changes can lead to incontinence, infections, and difficult intercourse (herbs and exercises help prevent such miseries); heart disease rates increase (Wise Woman ways can greatly reduce your risk); bones can lose density (simple foods and herbs can halt and reverse osteoporosis); joints act up; and wrinkles grow deeper.

With the help of home remedies, herbal allies, and Grandmother Growth's wise words, your post-menopausal years can be vital and beautiful. Remember, the *ugly* old woman/witch is the invention of male-dominant cultures, and our own fear of death. In peaceful matrifocal cultures, the beauty of crones is legendary: old women are satin-skinned, softly wrinkled, silver-haired, and awe-inspiring in their truth and dignity.

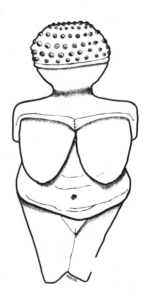

# Vaginal/Bladder Changes

*"Mother woman, you flowed, you flowed," sings Grandmother Growth.*
*"In rich fertility you flowed. You flowed with blood. You flowed*
*with fertility. As Mother, you flowed with milk, with life.*
*"Crone woman's blood does not flow. Crone woman's womb bears*
*no children, her breasts fill no more with milk. Are her flowing days*
*over? Not so, not so. Your flow has not ended, young Crone. Your flow*
*has gone underground. Your flow is held inside.*
*"Listen carefully, great granddaughter. When your wise blood stays*
*inside, it may make your belly heavy, hot, and dry. To keep your uterus,*
*vagina, and bladder soft and moist, you need to keep your wise blood*
*circulating and your root energies moving. Let the belly relax and sag a*
*bit so the blood and energy can move freely. Take time to be with yourself*
*sensuously, pleasurably, lovingly, stirring the cauldron of your belly and*
*the fires at your root. Take time to listen to the memories released when*
*the wise blood is kept flowing and spiraling inside your belly. Listen to*
*your inner stirrings. Stir the energy in your root chakra, and spiral it up*
*to sparkle at the crown. Then, listen, listen, listen."*

The pelvic (root) energies of the post-menopausal woman, having
no outlet in menstruation or birth, easily become congested. This
congestion traps hot energies in the vagina, bladder, uterus, and anus,
reducing vaginal lubrication, thinning and irritating the vagina and
vulva (vaginal lips), instigating constipation, encouraging incontinence,
and giving rise to vaginal atrophy and chronic vaginal yeast and bladder
infections.

Thinning and drying of pelvic tissues can occur rapidly (within 6-10
months of the last menses) when menopause is induced, the adrenals/
kidneys are weak, or there is insufficient body weight.

Women who achieve menopause naturally, carry enough body fat,
and nourish their adrenals/kidneys, will experience few problems with
vaginal/bladder weakness in the post-menopausal years.

## Dry Vagina

*"You have been wet and fertile at the will and whim of your body for*
*most of your years, great granddaughter," murmurs Grandmother*
*Growth. "But you have Changed. You grow moist with readiness for*
*play now only when you truly desire it, not at reproduction's dictates.*
*Have no fear that your springs have run dry. If you consciously call up*

*your flood of pleasure, it will answer. This is one of my greatest gifts to you, young Crone. No longer will you be accessible to those who do not inspire love and trust in you. The great portals of life, your womb, your vagina, now serve only you, now open only at your bidding."*

### Step 1. Collect information . . .

We are given two contradictory pictures of post-menopausal sex. On one hand, we're to look forward to freedom from conception worries, resulting in more spontaneous, relaxed, joyful sex filled with multiple orgasms. On the other hand, we're to expect dried-up, atrophied vaginas and dyspareunia (painful intercourse).

Thinning and drying of the vaginal tissues in the post-menopausal years is often first noticed during sexual activity when the expected lubrication is slight or absent. Is this normal? Are you a dried up old woman?

Yes, it is normal; almost all post-menopausal women will experience a lessening of sexual lubrication. No, you don't have to give up your sexual self. Crones know there are many ways to ecstasy besides intercourse, and many ways to get slippery when we want to.

(Extreme thinning and drying of the vagina is discussed on page 133.)

### Step 2. Engage the energy . . .

• **Homeopathic remedies** include:

☞ *Bryonia:* root chakra overheated and dry, dry vagina, dry stools/constipation.

☞ *Lycopodium:* lack of root stability, vagina very dry, self-confidence withered, skin dry.

☞ *Belladonna:* vagina painfully dry and too sensitive to tolerate touch.

• This yoga posture sounds simple, but requires concentration. Squeeze the anal/pelvic floor muscles firmly while inhaling; hold. Breathe out, holding the root lock and add a chin lock. Hold for two seconds. Visualize the nectar of the universe flowing down your spine and between your legs. Relax as you inhale.

★ **Slowly, slowly.** Give yourself plenty of time to warm up before inserting anything into your vagina.

### Step 3. Nourish and tonify . . .

★ **Comfrey root sitz bath** is an old favorite for keeping vaginal tissues flexible, strong, and soft. Brew up two quarts/liters of the infusion, rewarm, strain, and "sitz" in it for 5-10 minutes several times a week.

• Drink more water, not more tea or coffee or juice or soda . . . **water**. Or boil a small handful of rice in sixteen ounces/500 ml or more of water to make a thin broth regarded as an ideal internal moistener for women with dry vaginal tissues or dry mouths. Drink freely.

★ As part of your love play, chew on a small piece of **Dang Gui** root. It is said to increase vaginal lubrication.

• Pause for the soothing cooling touch of **chickweed** tincture, 25-40 drops in water, several times a day for 2-4 weeks, and see if your hot, dry vaginal tissues don't smile moistly.

• Increase vaginal lubrication and the thickness of your vaginal walls by starting your day with one of these remedies: 25 drops of **motherwort** tincture or 1-3 teaspoonfuls/5-15 ml of **safflower** or **flax** seed oil. Look for results within a month.

★ **Acidophilus capsules inserted vaginally** help prevent yeast infections and create copious amounts of lubrication. Insert one (or two) about 4-6 hours before lovemaking.

★ **Comfrey** ointment is the ally of choice when skin needs flexible strength. Rub in morning and night and use as a lubricant for love play. The vulva will be noticeably plumper and moister within three weeks.

• If you have access to **slippery elm**, try this soothing vaginal gel. Slowly heat 2 tablespoons/30ml slippery elm bark powder in a cup/250ml of water, stirring until thick. Cool (you can even chill it) before spreading over and inside the vulva and vagina. This gel lubricates, heals, and nourishes.

★ **Exercise, exercise.** Every part of your body will age more gracefully if you work it out regularly. That goes for your vagina and vulva, too. Weekly orgasm is the recommended exercise, but daily **pelvic floor exercises** tonify the vaginal tissues, too. See box, page 134.

### Step 4. Stimulate/Sedate . . .

• Avoid the problem of scanty lubrication: Try sensual, sexual excitations that don't involve intercourse.

★ Ointment made from **wild yam** roots may be the herbal equivalent of estrogen cream in its ability to restore youthful moistness and elasticity to post-menopausal vaginal tissues.

• You are more likely to be troubled by vaginal dryness and loss of lubrication if your adrenals have been exhausted by overuse of coffee, alcohol, and white sugar; severe stress; or dependence on steroid/ cortisone drugs.

• Herbalist Rina Nissim suggests applying the essential oil of *Salvia sclarea* to vaginal tissues that have lost their elasticity. Dilute with olive oil; pure essential oils can be fierce on sensitive mucus surfaces.

### Step 5a. Use supplements . . .

• Daily doses of 100-600 IU of vitamin E for 4-6 weeks can help you increase vaginal lubrication. You may need to continue with your daily dose for months to maintain your juiciness. Experiment to find the lowest effective dose for you. (See cautions, page 62.)

### Step 5b. Use drugs . . .

• Polycarbophil, the active ingredient in Replens (an over-the-counter cream) pulls water into vaginal cells, helping restore and maintain healthy lubrication. It also increases alkalinity in the vagina, stepping up the natural resistance to vaginal infections.

• Estrogen creams really do revitalize vaginal tissue. But estrogen applied vaginally is absorbed by the blood and carries the same risks as estrogen taken orally. Occasional rather than regular use minimizes side effects.

★ **Progesterone creams** appear to be as effective as estrogen creams in restoring lubrication and to cause fewer side effects.

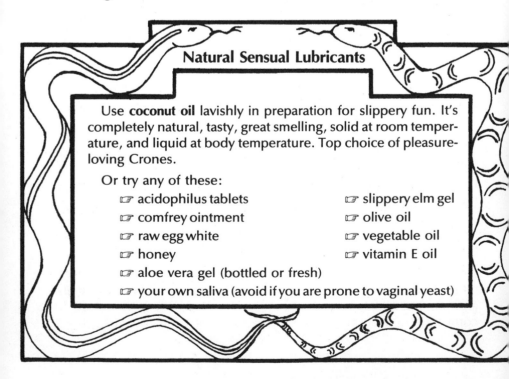

## Natural Sensual Lubricants

Use **coconut oil** lavishly in preparation for slippery fun. It's completely natural, tasty, great smelling, solid at room temperature, and liquid at body temperature. Top choice of pleasure-loving Crones.

Or try any of these:

☞ acidophilus tablets            ☞ slippery elm gel

☞ comfrey ointment            ☞ olive oil

☞ raw egg white            ☞ vegetable oil

☞ honey            ☞ vitamin E oil

☞ aloe vera gel (bottled or fresh)

☞ your own saliva (avoid if you are prone to vaginal yeast)

## Itching, Burning Vulva/Vaginal Atrophy

*"Do you feel like you're sitting on a vol . . . cane . . . ohhhhhhh!?" Grand-mother Growth's voice rises shrilly. "Who said Crones weren't hot?! Root chakra energies — anger, sex, power — are hot subjects. And this Change you call menopause fires the root chakra. Can you sit still in the midst of this rapidly vibrating energy? Can you run or dance with its searing touch? Oh granddaughter, what are you itching to do now that you are crowned Crone? What lights your passion? Shine, young Crone. Burn. And keep that energy stirred so your inner heat doesn't dry you out."*

### Step 1. Collect information . . .

Post-menopausal vaginal or vulval burning and itching is disrespect-fully labeled "senile vaginitis," "atrophic vaginitis," "vulvar dystrophy," or "atrophic vulvitis." (Also leukoplakia, lichen sclerosis, kraurosis, and sclerotic dermatosis.) This painful itching and burning (referred to as "pruritus" in premenopausal women) is caused by irritating, alkaline vaginal secretions acting on tender vaginal tissues. It is especially bothersome when the vaginal tissues are thin, dry, and cracked.

The following remedies stop the itching and burning and heal the crone's sensitive vagina/vulva (which may appear white, shiny, and clearly abraded or scratched), restoring pinkness, plumpness, and plia-bility, so long as there are no yeast overgrowths or bacterial infections to complicate the picture. (See pages 136-139 for yeast remedies.)

### Step 2. Engage the energy . . .

• Relax. Lie down. Watch your breath. See yourself breathing out through your vagina. Visualize yourself breathing cool blue energy in and out.

• **Homeopathic remedies** include:
   ☞ *Belladonna:* painful, hot vagina, tender, reddened.
   ☞ *Cantharis:* vagina burning and raw.
   ☞ *Sulfur:* vaginal itching is intense.
   ☞ *Natrum mur.:* the entire vagina, inside and out, is intensely painful.

### Step 3. Nourish and tonify . . .

★ **Motherwort** tincture (10-20 drops several times a day) quickly restores thickness and moisture to vaginal walls. So does regular use of **chaste tree**.

★ I've never met a crone's itch that could hold its own against **plantain** oil or ointment. Relief is immediate; the effect generally lasts for hours. Continued applications strengthen the skin, hasten healing, discourage infection, and stop inflammation. (See Appendix 2.)

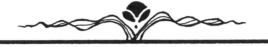

# Pelvic Floor Exercises (Kegels)

*Begin with fewer repetitions and gradually increase.*
*Expect results within 4-6 weeks.*

◇ While not usually considered an exercise, **sexual excitement** and orgasm is the best way to keep the vagina and vulva well nourished and well lubricated. Sexually active women actually have plumper, thicker cells in their bladders and vaginas than celibate women. Don't worry about having a partner; self-love is just fine for this remedy.

◇ To **increase vaginal lubrication**: Breathe out and push down as though you were trying to push something out of your vagina. Hold for 3 seconds. Inhale and relax. Do 25-50 repetitions.

◇ To **tone vaginal muscles** and increase lubrication: Tighten the inner muscles of the vagina tightly around a finger or small smooth marble or crystal egg and hold for up to 10-13 seconds; pulse (contract and relax) your vaginal muscles rapidly (10-30 times) as you breathe out. Repeat 10-25 times.

◇ To **tone vagina and bladder**: Sit in a basin or bathtub with water up to your hips. See if you can suck water into your vagina and expel it. Suck in as you breathe in; push out as you breathe out. Do 20-50 times.

◇ To **identify and strengthen the muscles that control voiding**: Next time you pee, stop the flow. Hold as long as you can (work up to at least ten seconds) before letting go and peeing again. As soon as you can, stop and hold again. Practice this every time you urinate.

◇ To **improve bladder control**: Pulse your urine flow by pushing the flow out very strongly, then slackening it off until it barely dribbles out, then push out strongly again, and again slack off. As a variation, push out strongly and increase the flow powerfully, then shut it off completely; repeat as many times as possible each time you urinate.

• Brew a quart/liter of **nettle** infusion several times a week. To thicken and nourish vaginal tissues, drink it or sit in it.

• **Calendula** cream applied morning and night helps strengthen vaginal tissues, heal minor abrasions, relieve pain, and discourage infection. So does **aloe vera gel**.

### Step 4. Sedate/Stimulate . . .

★ Take the time to sooth your vulva and yourself with an **oat bath**. Regular use encourages healthier tissues.

★ If there are no oats in the cupboard and the itching is driving you crazy, maybe there's some **honey**. Hygroscopic (water-drawing) honey will moisturize and heal your tender vulva. Apply directly where needed or pour some honey on a menstrual pad and wear it.

★ A **comfrey root** or **chamomile blossom** compress will soothe itchy, dry vaginal tissues and promote healthy skin growth. Infuse the comfrey root and soak a towel in the liquid. Or make a cup of camomile tea and use the teabag (warm, room temperature, or chilled). Apply either compress to your tenderness while in a reclining position.

• Massage in small circles around the inner and outer sides of your ankle bone to stimulate the flow of energy to the pelvic organs.

• Soap, douches, bubblebaths, nylon underwear, and pantyhose encourage itching/burning of the vagina/vulva.

### Step 5a. Use supplements . . .

★ Progesterone, especially that naturally derived from **wild yam roots** (*Dioscorea* species), applied directly to the vagina and vulva, is remarkably effective — results are often seen within days — but not curative. Discontinuing the progesterone ointment leads to recurrence of the burning and itching. In many cases, however, progesterone ointment helped women unaffected by estrogen or testosterone creams.

★ Daily ingestion of oils rich in omega-3 fatty acids (such as flax seed) can reverse vaginal thinning and drying, relieve itching and burning.

• Vitamin $B_2$ supplements may be helpful in relieving crone's itch.

### Step 5b. Use drugs . . .

• Natural or synthetic estrogen or testosterone creams are used to remedy very thin, irritated vaginal tissues. To minimize increased cancer risk, use a very small amount (say, ⅛ applicator) only as needed.

• Vaginal anti-itch creams containing cortisone may be used as a last resort, cortisone contributes to osteoporosis.

# Vaginal Yeast Overgrowth

*"Old sour puss, they used to call the spinster." Grandmother Growth closes her eyes and a sly grin spreads over her face. "Well, I guess a crone has a right to a sour puss, sure enough. That way she doesn't wind up scratching her privates in public."*

### Step 1. Collect information . . .

Yeast (*Candida albicans* or *monilia*) is a natural part of a healthy vaginal environment. It helps prevent the growth of infective bacteria.

If the yeast grows too much, it is noticeable as a nice-smelling, white, cottage-cheese-like accumulation on your vaginal walls or in your underwear. Yeast overgrowth can make your vagina and vulva very irritated, sensitive, sore, and itchy, and can even cause episodes of incontinence.

Lactobacilli such as acidophilus are also residents of a healthy vagina. They prevent yeast overgrowths. They also turn milk into yogurt. Lactobacilli thrive when your vagina is acidic. When vaginal acidity drops, yeasts thrive.

You can check the pH of your vagina with litmus paper. A healthy acidic reading would be 4 to 4.5. Yeast overgrowth begins at 5.5 and irritation is usually evident when the pH reaches 6 or higher (more alkaline).

As estrogen and progesterone stop stimulating the reproductive tissues, vaginal secretions naturally become less acidic and yeast overgrowths are more common. When the **Change** is rapid (as in induced menopause), the upsurge in vaginal yeast causes incredibly intense itching. When the **Change** is slower, the lactobacilli have time to adapt to the less acidic environment and yeast overgrowth is minimized.

Post-menopausal women choosing ERT/HRT are often bothered with vaginal yeast overgrowths, as are diabetic crones, and those who must take frequent antibiotics.

These tried-and-trusted remedies, from the grandmothers and wise women of today and yesterday, offer fast, effective relief. Note: If you experience chronic or repeated vaginal yeast overgrowths, all of your love play partners need to use remedies, too, not just you.

### Step 2. Engage the energy . . .

★ What is the benefit of a vaginal yeast overgrowth? Many women say it gives them an excuse to say **"No"** to sex. Here are some other ways to say it:

☞ Stand in front of a mirror and say "No" at least 25 times.

☞ Yell "No" and stamp your foot ten times. Breathe.
☞ Stand in front of your lover. Keep your eyes open. Say "No."
☞ Hold your arms at shoulder level, palms out, push against a tree or a wall or the palms of another person, and say "No!"

**Step 3. Nourish and tonify . . .**

★ Insert one or two capsules of **acidophilus powder** into your vagina every other day for two weeks. Acidophilus is a variety of lactobacillus. If you keep adding lactobacilli to the vagina, the yeast stops growing. Be sure to push the capsule all the way up to the cervix (feels like the tip of your nose).

• If the yeast is persistent, insert the acidophilus capsule *behind* the cervix, in the little pocket between it and the vaginal wall nearest the rectum. (Putting one foot up on a chair, while standing on the other, helps open the vagina and ease insertion.) And **treat all your play partners**, too. Have male partners soak their members in apple cider vinegar or diluted yogurt for five minutes daily to kill yeast living in and on the glans.

• Other ways to nourish lactobacilli (to the detriment of the yeast):
☞ Eat a cup of **plain yogurt** daily.
☞ Insert 1-2 tablespoons/15-30 ml of plain yogurt in the vagina every day or so. (Be imaginative, you *can* get it in there.)
☞ Use a yogurt sitz bath. (Dilute 16 ounces/125 ml yogurt in 2 quarts/500 ml warm water.)

★ Make sure your yogurt contains live cultures (it will say on the label). If it does, your symptoms will usually be relieved within 48 hours.

• Sweets of any kind (sugar, fruit juices, even artificial sweeteners) can change the vaginal pH enough to encourage yeast overgrowth, especially in the post-menopausal years.

★ "So long as I drink my 2 cups of **nettle** infusion daily, my crotch feels fine, no itching, no burning, no yeast."

**Step 4. Stimulate/Sedate . . .**

• If neither acidophilus nor yogurt curbs your yeast overgrowth, try these ways to reacidify your vagina (in order of increasing strength):
☞ **Apple cider vinegar:** Use 4 tablespoons/60 ml in a quart/liter of water as a sitz bath or douche, once or twice daily. Results evident in 3 days; continue for 10 days. Or alternate with acidophilus every other day for a week.
☞ **White vinegar (acetic acid):** Use 1 tablespoon/15 ml in a quart/liter of water. Sitz or douche as above.

☞ **Lemon juice**: same as for white vinegar.
☞ **Lactic acid** (sold as Lactinex powder): as directed.
☞ **Boric acid**: a heavy-duty measure. Have the druggist put 600 mg boric acid in 00 gelatin caps (or fill them yourself). Insert one high up in the vagina, by the cervix, every day or so for two weeks.

★ If yeast remedies work, but only temporarily, there are probably bacteria as well as yeast thriving in the vagina. Bacteria create the alkaline conditions that yeast love. No matter how acidic you make your vagina, the bacteria undo all your efforts and soon the yeast is growing again. **To eliminate mild bacterial infections**, insert a clove of garlic high up in the vagina, on or behind the cervix, before going to bed every night for 5-10 days. CAUTION: Tender tissues may be burned by garlic juice, so peel the clove gently, don't crush. Generously grease and/or wrap the garlic in thin material before inserting. Note: Your breath and sweat will smell of garlic if you use this remedy.

• Vaginal penetration in love play when there's a yeast overgrowth causes friction which irritates the vaginal walls and makes the overgrowth more difficult to remedy.

• Yeast loves the hot, moist environment of pantyhose, nylon underwear, swimsuits, tight pants.

• Bubblebath, douches, and soap make the vaginal environment more alkaline, that is, more friendly to yeast. Women who douche more than three times a month are 4-5 times more likely to have vaginal yeast overgrowths.

• Crones may want to avoid using goldenseal or myrrh douches (often recommended to remedy chronic vaginal yeast overgrowth). Both of these herbs are quite drying.

*Step 5a. Use supplements . . .*

• High doses of vitamin B complex may help remedy chronic vaginal yeast overgrowths. Note that daily consumption of nutritional yeast (often recommended as a source of B vitamins) can leach calcium from the bones.

*Step 5b. Use drugs . . .*

• **Gentian violet** is a dangerous, concentrated fungicide (yeast killer) despite its innocent name. It is very messy, but very effective. Use cotton swabs to paint a one percent aqueous solution on the cervix, vaginal walls, and vulva before going to bed. Wear a sanitary pad to contain the staining. Repeat 4-6 times during the next 2 weeks.

CAUTION: If this causes burning, immediately insert some plain yogurt into your vagina or sit in a tub of vinegared water.

• Nystatin (Nilstat or Mycostatin) is also a fungicide. Yeast infections often recur after a nystatin cure.

• Stronger drugs include miconazole (Monistat) and clotrimazole (Gyne-Lotrimin). Metronidazole (Flagyl), taken orally, may be prescribed when the infection is severe and chronic. CAUTION: Flagyl causes gene mutations and cancer in animal studies. Recent studies with women implicate Flagyl as a *cause* of yeast overgrowth and a contributor to depression.

# Incontinence

*"A sour puss, a crazy lady, and a real pisser, yep, that's me," Grandmother Growth declares with mischief in her sparkling eyes. "And if you don't want to wet your pants, young Crone, come close. Let me teach you how to stir your fluids so they don't leak out at inopportune moments."*

### Step 1. Collect information

Most women (65-75 percent) will experience one or more occurrences of stress and/or urge incontinence in the decades following menopause.

Stress incontinence refers to urine leakage when the bladder is stressed. Stresses include laughing, sneezing, coughing, picking something up, running, and other normal activities that put stress on the bladder.

Urge incontinence refers to urine leakage as soon as the urge to void is felt, with no time to remove clothing or find a toilet

The known causes of stress and urge incontinence include: weakened or damaged pelvic floor from pelvic surgery (including caesarean section and hysterectomy), precipitous birth, repeated pregnancies; thinning bladder wall after menopause; medications (both prescription and over-the-counter); frequent use of alcohol; urinary tract infections; fibroids; and constipation. Isolated incidents of incontinence are usually due to bacteria in the bladder or lack of tone in the pelvic muscles and bladder, and are easily remedied. The following remedies are helpful for women with chronic incontinence, as well.

### Step 2. Engage the energy . . .

• **Homeopathic** remedies include:
  ☞ *Pulsatilla*: bladder and pelvic floor feel unreliable or weak.
  ☞ *Zincum met.*: there is frequent slight loss of urine.

★ **Biofeedback** is an excellent way for the woman with incontinence to learn to pinpoint and control the muscles of her bladder and urethra. Controlled scientific studies show a success rate of 55-80 percent with twice-daily use of a biofeedback machine. You can buy biofeedback machines or go to a clinic to use one. The ultimate biofeedback machine, of course, is your own body and its sensory abilities.

★ **Empty** the bladder *completely* every time you void by pressing down behind your pubic bone with fingertips or flat of your palm. This can be a critical move in changing your relationship with your bladder.

### Step 3. Nourish and tonify . . .

★ Boil dried **teasel** (*Dipsacus sylvestris*) roots, a tablespoon to a cup/250 ml of water for ten to fifteen minutes, and drink daily to strengthen and restore tone to overstretched sphincter muscles. This is a favored and specific cure for incontinence.

★ It's all in the timing. One of the most effective remedies for occasional and even chronic incontinence is **scheduled toileting.** Go to the toilet on a regular schedule, say every 60-90 minutes. After 3-4 consecutive dry days, increase the interval by 15-30 minutes, and continue increasing until you can handle intervals of four hours or more.

• Some women report a daily eye-opener of **cranberry juice** helps relieve urge incontinence.

★ Urge and stress incontinence, even when caused by surgical damage or post-menopausal thinning of the bladder walls, are lessened noticeably when you commit yourself to **pelvic floor exercises.** Like any tonic, they give the best effect when done regularly and repeatedly for months or years. See page 134.

### Step 4. Sedate/Stimulate . . .

★ Push hard on the very top of the head to relieve urge incontinence on the spot.

• **Antispasmodic herbs** such as black cohosh, ginger, catnip, and cornsilk may help when incontinence comes from a hyperactive bladder (more frequent with urge incontinence than stress incontinence). Use 10-20 drops of **black cohosh** tincture once or twice daily for several weeks or as needed. A tea of any of the others may be taken freely. **Ginger** will warm and help relieve constipation (which may contribute to urge incontinence). **Catnip** is so relaxing that it can be sleep-inducing. **Cornsilk** is an excellent herb for strengthening the bladder and removing minor infections; however, it is also a diuretic, which might cancel its benefits for some women.

• Caffeine, alcohol, and white sugar aggravate both stress incontinence and urge incontinence in many women. Other common bladder irritants include: citrus, tomatoes, cayenne, hot peppers, iced drinks or very cold foods, pineapple, and carbonated drinks.

• Regular use of tobacco increases your risk of developing stress incontinence by 350 percent.

• The **water cure** aims to pump energy into the pelvic floor and strengthen the bladder. Set out two shallow basins: one with very hot water and one with icy cold water. Start by relaxing for three minutes in the hot one. Then lower yourself up and down, in and out of the icy water for one minute. Repeat 3-4 times; do it several times a week. (My mother would call this the kind of remedy where the cure is worse than the problem!)

• For those who cannot for the life of them figure out which muscles are weak and causing their incontinence, seek out the Physiostim machine. It contracts your pelvic floor muscles with electrical stimulation. Then you try to duplicate the motion yourself while a biofeedback machine tells you how close you're getting.

*Step 5a. Use supplements . . .*

★ Progesterone creams, such as those made from **wild yam** roots, are used vaginally to help restore healthy tone to bladder tissues.

*Step 5b. Use drugs . . .*

• Many common prescription and non-prescription drugs can provoke incontinence, including diuretics, antidepressants, beta-blockers, the popular high-blood-pressure drug Minipress (prazosin), sleeping pills, tranquilizers, and urinary tract anti-infectives.

• ERT/HRT and estrogen vaginal creams are highly effective at reversing incontinence caused by vaginal and bladder wall thinning.

*Step 6. Break and enter . . .*

• Surgery is a highly publicized, but risky and invasive cure for incontinence. In one study, 25 percent of the women had no improvement after surgery. Another 25 percent improved only slightly. And half of the women could not empty their bladders at all after the surgery (slight overcorrection there) and had to learn to catheterize themselves.

• Hysterectomy is not a cure for incontinence.

*"Having experienced episodes of urge incontinence all my life, I have watched carefully to see what triggers them. And for me it is clearly linked with sub-clinical urinary tract infections. So long as I'm totally infection-free, I don't go until I'm ready to go."*

# Bladder Infections

*"If you let that fiery wise blood just sit there in your belly, great grand-daughter," admonishes Grandmother Growth, "you'll get the urge to quench that heat. You'll get a tickle, a twinge, an urgent call. But you won't have the moisture you need. It's boiled away. It's gone up in steam.*

*"So I'll say it once more: circulate your wise blood, granddaughter. Spiral it around and up to your crown. Take action on your anger. Pleasure yourself. And you'll be one of those old crones, like me, whose eyes sparkle with mirth and flash with intention."*

### Step 1. Collect information . . .

Bladder infections are also known as cystitis, urethritis, and UTIs (urinary tract infections). When bacteria grow in the bladder, the resulting infection usually causes symptoms such as: a burning sensation during voiding, overwhelming urgency, frequent but minuscule urinations, incontinence, bloody urine, and pelvic pain. But up to 25 percent of the bladder infections in post-menopausal women are silent or symptomless.

Bacteria enter the bladder in three primary ways: when feces are spread to the bladder opening (such as wiping from back to front after toileting), when the tube leading to the bladder is irritated or bruised (as from use of a diaphragm, pelvic surgery, or prolonged/vigorous vaginal penetration), or when there is an in-dwelling catheter. The thinning and shrinking of reproductive and bladder tissues that may occur in the post-menopausal years contributes to bladder infections in older women, as does lessening of vaginal acidity. In addition, tiny ulcerations of the bladder may occur, usually in the absence of infection; this is called interstitial cystitis (IC). The remedies gathered here are substantially the same ones that have delighted and aided the readers of my *Wise Woman Herbal for the Childbearing Year*. Note that only a few of these remedies are beneficial for women with interstitial cystitis and some are contraindicated for such women.

### Step 2. Engage the energy . . .

★ **Flow, flow, flow.** Head off that bladder infection by drinking a glass of water hourly as soon as you feel the first urgency or burning. It is tempting to stint on drinking if you find yourself unexpectedly incontinent, but don't. Bladder infections only make incontinence worse.

• Urine is ideally neutral to slightly acidic (pH 5.8 – pH 7). Very acidic urine (below pH 5.5) encourages infections. An established infection gives rise to alkaline urine (pH 7.5 or higher) which causes stinging and burning. Test your urine with pH paper any time *except* first thing in the morning. You can use cranberry juice to lower the pH; vitamin C to raise it.

• *Cantharis* is a homeopathic remedy for scalding urine.

### Step 3. Nourish and tonify . . .

• **Cranberries** (*Vaccinium macrocarpon*) contain substances that kill bacteria *and* make your bladder wall so slippery that any escaping bacteria can't latch on and thrive there. Unsweetened cranberry juice (or concentrate) is the most effective form. (The sugar or corn syrup in cranberry cocktail-type juices and cran-apple juices can feed the infection.) Drink freely, at least a glass a day, up to a quart/liter a day for acute infections unless your urine's pH is already low.

★ Pelvic floor exercises even help prevent and relieve bladder infections! See page 134 and try this one: After urinating, close your eyes, relax, breathe out, and see if you can squeeze out an extra dribble.

• **Mallows** of any kind make a delightfully soothing infusion for irritated bladders. Marsh mallow (*Althea officinalis*) is the classic, but I've also used *Malva sylvestris, rotundifolia,* and *neglecta.* Soak a small handful of the fresh root or 2 tablespoonfuls/15 grams of the dried in 8 ounces/60 ml water overnight; strain and drink next morning. This remedy is one of the best for women with IC.

• Another remedy for women with IC: Cook one cup/250 ml barley in 8 cups/2 liters water until soft. Drink 1 cup/250 ml at least every other day for a month or more. Expect fast, soothing results.

• An overgrowth of vaginal yeast may be irritating your bladder or urethra. Eat one cup of plain yogurt 4-5 times a week.

### Step 4. Sedate/Stimulate . . .

★ **Uva Ursi** (*Arctostaphylos uva ursi*) is an old favorite for strengthening the bladder and ending chronic silent bladder infections. I prefer the hot water infusion of the dried leaves, but have heard from women successfully using cold water infusions or tinctures with vodka or vinegar. Dose is 1 cup/125 ml of infusion or 2 teaspoons/10 ml of vinegar or 10 drops of tincture, 3-6 times a day initially, then 1-3 times a day for 7-10 days. In very chronic cases, eliminate of all forms of sugar (even fresh fruit, fruit juice, and honey) for a month as well.

★ **Yarrow** is a urinary disinfectant with a powerful antibacterial action and an astringent effect wonderful for shaping up weak, lax bladder tissues. Use a small cup of the infusion once or twice a day for 7-10 days, or combine it half and half with uva ursi. Results may be felt within several hours. Highly recommended for women with IC.

★ In my experience, *Echinacea purpurea* and *E. augustifolia* are as effective as antibiotics in clearing bladder infections and do *not* contribute to vaginal yeast. (See step 5b.) I use a dose of 1 drop echinacea tincture per 2 pounds/1 kilo body weight. (For 150 pound/70 kilo person, use 75 drops or three dropperfuls.) In acute cases, I give the dose every 2 hours. As the infection clears, I lengthen the amount of time between doses until I'm down to 1-2 doses a day, which I continue for another 2-10 weeks.

• Women who wash their vulva with soap and water are four times *more* likely to get vaginal and bladder infections. Women who use diaphragms are 2-4 times more likely to get bladder infections. Douches, bubblebaths, tampons, nylon underwear, and pantyhose may also irritate the urethra and contribute to bladder infections.

• Known bladder irritants include: alcohol, black tea, coffee, sodas, citrus juices, chocolate, cayenne, and hot peppers. (An herbal tincture in an alcohol base won't irritate the bladder if you take it diluted in a glass of water or cup of herb tea.) Women with IC, pay close attention to this list.

• **Urinating after love play** flushes out bacteria and cuts down on UTIs. Urinating before love play, however, increases your risk of a bladder infection.

• Acupuncture has been an effective remedy for some women with IC.

*Step 5a. Use supplements . . .*

• The addition of 1-3 tablespoons/15-45 ml of **flax seed oil** to the diet has been effective in relieving chronic bladder infections.

• Ascorbic acid (vitamin C) wrings the kidneys, flushes the bladder, and raises urinary pH. Try 500 mg hourly for 6-8 hours.

• Be careful about taking calcium supplements if you are prone to bladder infections. Calcium supplements increase bacterial adherence to the bladder wall, thus greatly increasing bladder infections.

*Step 5b. Use drugs . . .*

• Antibiotics are the standard medical treatment for bladder infections. But taking antibiotics frequently causes vaginal yeast overgrowth (which can lead to a bladder infection). One antibiotic, nitrofurantoin (Macrodantin), seems to cause microscopic scarring and ulceration of the bladder wall, precipitating IC.

*Step 6. Break and enter...*

• Dilation of the urethra is expensive, painful, and causes tiny scars on the urethra which may lead to interstitial cystitis. I have seen it referred to as "the rape of the female urethra." No controlled study has shown this procedure to be effective at limiting chronic bladder infections. Do pelvic floor exercises instead. (See box, page 134.)

# Dry Mouth

*"Yes, you must learn to spit it out, great granddaughter. Say it out loud, sing it, express it for all to hear," says Grandmother Growth, licking her lips. "What? Mouth dry with stage fright? Chew this over with me, young Crone. Loosen your lips (speak your heart), expand your tongue (learn another language) and find the strength in your jaw (stand up for your rights). Is your mouth moist now?"*

*Step 1. Collect information...*

Dry mouth is not caused by aging. Salivary gland function remains strong in healthy people, no matter what their age. However, dry mouth may be a temporary problem during the menopausal years.

Decreased saliva production is a minor annoyance but a major health hazard. Without adequate saliva, teeth and gum tissues quickly become abraded, infected, and demineralized. As oral health declines, so does the ability to take in adequate nourishment. Use these remedies to help prevent such problems in your Crone years.

*Step 2. Engage the energy...*

• Fear is the emotion connected with dry mouth. (See pages 81-85.) Remember that fear is the messenger of hidden desires.

*Step 3. Nourish and tonify...*

★ Drink rice or barley water. Boil a handful of grain in 4 cups/1000 ml water for an hour. These soothing grain beverages nourish deeply, supporting the body's ability to keep the mouth moist.

• Sip nourishing and soothing herbal brews such as **sassafras** leaf tea, **violet** leaf infusion, **marsh mallow** root tea, or **comfrey** leaf infusion throughout the day.

• Begin your day with a bowl of mouth-watering **oatmeal** and **slippery elm**. Replace up to 1 tablespoon/15 ml of 1/2 cup/125 ml dry oatmeal with slippery elm bark powder before cooking in 2 cups/500 ml water.

### Step 4. Stimulate/Sedate . . .

★ The easiest way to stimulate and encourage saliva production is to suck or chew on something. Try slippery elm lozenges, malt-sweetened hard candies (available in health food stores), or a piece of Dang Gui or licorice root (not licorice candy).

• Smoking slows saliva output; so does consumption of alcohol.

• Massage under the jaw, along the center of the bone, to relieve spasms in salivary glands.

### Step 5a. Use supplements . . .

• Dry mouth is related to deficiencies of iron, calcium, potassium, and B$_6$.

### Step 5b. Use drugs . . .

★ Medications are the major cause of dry mouth. Nearly 400 commonly prescribed drugs — including antihistamines, decongestants, anti-depressants, and high blood pressure medicines — list dry mouth as a side effect. With the exception of licorice root, which may be contra-indicated for those taking blood pressure medicines, the remedies in steps 2, 3, and 4 are effective and safe to take with medications.

# Post-Menopausal Vaginal Bleeding

*"Crones hold their wise blood inside," declares Grandmother Growth. "Crones stir their wise blood inside. Your menses have stopped. Crones hold their wise blood inside."*

### Step 1. Collect information . . .

Vaginal bleeding in a post-menopausal woman is generally cause for alarm, but not for panic. There are a few benign causes: A sudden increase in optimum nutrition, such as the addition of nourishing herbal infusions to your diet, may tickle one or two last eggs into developing, causing a "normal" menstrual cycle. So can falling in love, they say. Blood spots during or after love play generally come from slight tears in more delicate older vaginal tissues or small cervical polyps (generally benign), commonly found among crones.

If you rule out these possibilities, seek help from someone experienced in women's health care.

## Post-Menopausal Vaginal/Bladder Changes
# References & Resources

pH paper (ColorpHast) by mail from EM Science, 111 Woodcrest Rd, Cherry Hill, NJ 08034 ($10)

Biofeedback equipment from Self Care Catalog, 5850 Shellmound Avenue, Emeryville, CA 94662-0813

"Chronic UTIs," National Women's Health Network News, May 1985 & Jan. 1987

"Chronic Vaginitis," Bobbie Hasselbring, Medical Self Care, Feb. 1988

Continence Restored, 407 Strawberry Hill Av, Stamford, CT 06902

Foundation for Continence, Box 835, Wilmette, IL 60091 • Info, support group contacts.

"Herbal/alternative management of urinary tract infections," Medical Herbalism, Fall 1991, POBox 33080, Portland, OR, 97233 ($5)

HIP: Help For Incontinent People, POBox 544, Union, SC 29379 • Audio tape and booklet on pelvic floor exercises; also, "Resource Guide for Continence Aids & Services" for $3.

"Home Remedies for Vaginitis," Santa Cruz Women's Health Center, 250 Locust St, Santa Cruz, CA 95060 ($.50 plus SASE)

"Incontinence," Hot Flash Newsletter, Vol. #5, No. 2

Interstitial Cystitis Association, POBox 4178, Great Neck, NY 11207

"Natural Healing in Gynecology," Rina Nissim, Pandora, 1984

"The New Healing Yourself," Joy Gardener, Crossing Press, 1989

"Overcoming Bladder Disorders," Rebecca Chalker & Kristene Whitmore, Harper, 1990 • Lots of home remedies; recommended.

"Topical progesterone in treatment of vulvar dystrophy," E. Jasionowski, MD, American Journal of Obstet. Gynecol. 127:667, 1977

"Urinary Incontinence in Adults," Office of Medical Applications of Research, Building 1, Room 260, Bethesda, MD 20892 • Free.

"Urinary Incontinence," in "Growing Older, Getting Better," Jane Porcino, Addison-Wesley, 1983

"UTIs," S. Hoffman, American Health, April 1989

"Vaginitis," Harvard Medical School Health Letter, Feb. 1984

"Wise Woman Herbal for the Childbearing Year," Susun Weed, Ash Tree, 1986

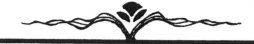

# Hypertension/High Blood Pressure

★ Deep relaxation and yoga breathing, such as alternate-nostril breath, calms the sympathetic nervous system, thus relaxing the small arteries, and permanently lowers blood pressure.

★ Use the tincture of **hawthorn, motherwort,** or **dandelion** to reduce hypertension, tonify your heart (and blood vessels), and eliminate excess fluid. Regular use for 2-3 months may be necessary before results are measurable. (These tonifying herbs literally rebuild your blood vessels and heart muscle, and that takes some time.)

★ **Potassium** is the critical mineral for maintenance of healthy blood pressure. The great majority of hypertensives (80-85 percent) who eat six portions of potassium-rich foods daily will reduce their need for medication by half or more. See Appendix 1 for sources of potassium.

★ Eat ½-1 clove of raw **garlic** a day and watch your blood pressure drop. My favorite raw garlic dishes:
  ☞ Scrambled eggs topped with minced raw garlic.
  ☞ Tomato sauce with chopped raw garlic added just before eating.
  ☞ Yogurt cheese with minced raw garlic on whole wheat crackers.
  ☞ Minced raw garlic on a baked potato.
  ☞ Herb vinegar and minced raw garlic on cooked greens like dandelion, nettles, spinach, kale, collards, mustard, amaranth, or lamb's quarters.

★ **Ginseng** is well documented as a highly effective blood pressure regulator. So is seaweed.

• Hypertensive medications lower blood pressure by draining fluids from circulation (diuretics) or by blocking the nerve signals that constrict the arteries (beta blockers). But diuretics may actually increase the risk of heart attack by leaching potassium salts needed by the heart; and the heart may respond to blocked nerve signals by trying harder, and harder, until it fails.

If you currently take blood pressure medications, and wish to experiment with easing off them, do it gradually, monitor your blood pressure several times a day, and use one or more of the above remedies for several weeks first.

• Note: Regular consumption of meat, coffee, table salt, and more than one alcoholic drink a day will raise your blood pressure. Vegetarians rarely have high blood pressure.

# Heart Healthy

*"Open your heart to me, my own," whispers Grandmother Growth so softly you aren't certain you hear her. "Open the wisdom way of compassion here in your heart and draw me inside. Let Grandmother Growth be inside you, helping you encompass the whole, in the beat of your heart, my heart, Crone's heart."*

### Step 1. Collect information . . .

You can hardly have escaped hearing that post-menopausal American women die from heart disease at rates as high as men's. (Women account for 51 percent of all cardiovascular deaths; men, 49 percent.) And that heart disease is America's top killer (claiming a life every 34 seconds). And that ERT will protect you. If avoidance of hot flashes isn't enough, isn't this an even stronger reason to take ERT? (HRT does not seem to prevent heart disease nearly as well as unopposed estrogen.)

It is not a given that estrogen protects your heart, however. In fact, it is well established that ERT raises blood pressure, increases the level of triglycerides, and increases blood clotting (leading to strokes). HRT has also been shown to increase risks of stroke and heart attack. Medical studies in the 1950s actually showed increases in heart disease and mortality with estrogen supplementation. I think it's singularly instructive that women whose ovaries are surgically removed at a young age (thus depriving them of estrogen and progesterone) do not have a higher incidence of heart attacks than other women their age.

Even if ERT/HRT does reduce death from cardiovascular causes, it nonetheless increases deaths from cancers of the breast and uterus. Advocates of ERT maintain that it saves more lives from heart disease than it takes with cancer, but this is only true if we assume that women are unwilling or unable to take care of themselves. **More than 90 percent of all heart disease is preventable with lifestyle changes.**

Crones can virtually eliminate heart disease by eating a low fat diet, stopping smoking, keeping blood pressure low, exercising regularly, practicing compassion, and gradually shedding truly excess weight — all goals easily achieved with Wise Woman ways. (The three top risk factors for women, vis-à-vis heart disease, are too much belly fat, smoking, and untreated hypertension. High cholesterol is one of the top three risk factors for men, but not for women.)

### Step 2. Engage the energy . . .

• **Rose** flower essence and rose quartz essence are both recommended for engaging the energy of the heart.

• Do you attack your heart? Do you close your heart to protect it? Love yourself. Give yourself plenty of nice strokes so you won't have a bad stroke. Try Stephen Levine's meditation on "Opening the Heart" in *Who Dies?* (Anchor, 1982).

• People in Hawaii, New Mexico, and Arizona have the lowest cardiovascular disease and coronary/stroke rates in the United States. Imagine you live there.

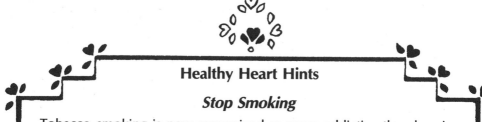

### Healthy Heart Hints

#### *Stop Smoking*

Tobacco smoking is now recognized as more addictive than heroin. To give you an extra edge while quitting, nourish yourself with a handful of **sunflower seeds** and a cup of **nettle** or **oatstraw** infusion daily for 4-6 weeks *before* quitting. Sunflower seeds reduce the body's craving for nicotine (by filling the nicotine receptor sites); the optimum nourishment from the herbal infusion strengthens the blood vessels and nerves and cushions the impact of withdrawal.

During your first 30 days off tobacco, try these Wise Woman ways:

◇ Take an oatstraw bath. (See Appendix 2.)

◇ Get a massage.

◇ Eat a wild salad (even if it's only one dandelion leaf).

◇ Bring home a flower.

◇ Ask someone to cook dinner for you.

◇ Go to a yoga class or a martial arts class (many places offer one free introductory class).

◇ Read the section on "Constipation" (pages 33-34), a frequent symptom of nicotine withdrawal.

◇ Buy yourself something extravagant with the money you would have spent on a month's worth of cigarettes.

◇ Take a break every time you would have smoked a cigarette and do something pleasurable.

◇ Affirm that it is better to gain 10-15 pounds/5-7 kilos than to die of lung cancer. Ex-smokers say the weight leaves after a year or two.

◇ Read, get, buy *The No-Nag, No-Guilt, Do-It-Your-Own-Way Guide to Quitting Smoking* by Tom Ferguson, MD, Ballantine, 1987.

*Step 3. Nourish and tonify . . .*

★ **Touch and be touched.** In numerous scientific studies, people who were touched lovingly every day had significantly fewer heart problems than the control groups.

★ **Hawthorn** berry tincture is the standard herbal heart tonic, and for good reason. It is broadly effective, virtually without overdose, and easy to make from fresh or dried berries. An elegant shrub or small tree, hawthorn is frequently cultivated in the suburbs. Injectable forms of *Crataegus* were used by MDs up until the 1950s to treat valvular heart disease, high blood pressure, inflammation of the heart muscle, and arteriosclerosis. The action of hawthorn is slow but complete. It strengthens the heart, establishes a regular heart beat, relieves water build-up around the heart, and resolves stress throughout the cardiovascular system. Dose is 25-40 drops of the berry tincture, up to 4 times a day. Expect results no sooner than 6-8 weeks.

★ Keep your heart healthy with regular use of **seaweeds**. Seaweeds have clinically proven cardiotonic effects: they stabilize blood pressure; regulate levels of triglycerides, phospholipids, and cholesterols (bad fats); dissolve fatty build-ups in the blood vessels; restore cardiac efficiency; prolong the life of the heart muscle; and encourage a steady heart beat. See my green book, *Healing Wise*, for delicious seaweed recipes.

• Women who eat foods rich in carotenes cut their risk of stroke by 40 percent. Foods rich in carotenes are those that are green, orange, yellow, and red. (See Appendix 1.)

★ **Garlic**, Knoblauch, Ail (*Allium sativum*) is a great friend to old hearts. Study after study has confirmed garlic's abilities to lower blood pressure, reduce phospholipids and cholesterol, strengthen heart action, increase immune response, reduce platelet clumping and clotting (thus reducing strokes), and stabilize blood sugar levels. Greatest benefit comes from ingesting it raw, or only lightly cooked, at least several cloves a day. (There are deodorized capsules that dissolve below your stomach so you can take lots without odorous burps.)

• **Essential fatty acids** are ever so essential to a healthy heart. Find them in wild foods, especially wild seeds such as **plantain, lamb's quarter,** and **amaranth** (*Plantago majus, Chenopodium album,* and *Amaranthus retroflexus*). Or in the fresh pressed oils of wheat germ, flax seed, borage seed, or black currant seed.

★ **Motherwort**, that dear friend of menopausal women, is a favorite heart tonic. A dose of 10-20 drops of the tincture of the flowering tops, taken up to three times a day, helps lower blood pressure, strengthen heart action, ease palpitations and irregular heart beats, and make room in the heart for compassion.

• **Lemon balm** is so strengthening to the heart that it is said that those who drink the tea daily will live forever. You can also steep a handful of fresh leaves in a glass of white wine for an hour or so and drink it with dinner. Or make lemon balm vinegar to use on your salads.

• You don't have to sweat, but you do have to **move!** to keep your heart healthy. Go for a walk, jump rope, swim, or do leg lifts and arm raises from your wheelchair or bed. However you can do it, do it.

## Healthy Heart Hints
### *Maintain a Healthy Weight*

Post-menopausal women nourish healthy hearts by making weight changes very slowly. Chinese herbalists consider it dangerous to the heart to *lose* weight after the age of forty. They point out that it is the diet as much as the excess weight that causes heart disease. "Eat right; do not worry about weight," sums up their attitude.

◇ **Up:** Post-menopausal women can continue a slow gain of ½ to 1 pound a year without increasing their risk of heart attack. (You don't have to weigh yourself. Take a pinch of belly fat: keep it under 2 inches and you're fine.)

◇ **Down:** Easiest way to lose weight? Just eliminate three things from your diet: meat, sugar, and white flour. Excess weight literally melts off with "no" effort. (That is, the only effort you have to make is to say "no.")

◇ **All over:** Restricted diets promote heart attacks. Frequent dieting, fasting, binging and purging unbalance your electrolyte levels, causing weakening of the heart muscle and damage to the heart. Infrequent bursts of exercise can also damage the heart and blood vessels.

◇ **Just right:** Eat as much as you want of whole grains, vegetables, beans, greens, fruits, fish, seeds, yogurt. Go easy on nuts, cheese, and milk. Drink water and herbal infusions as your beverages.

• **Dandelion root** tincture lowers blood pressure, reduces bad fats, and helps keep your heart and cardiovascular system healthy and happy. Use 10-15 drops with meals.

### Step 4. Sedate/Stimulate . . .

★ **Blood thinners**, like aspirin, reduce the incidence of strokes and diminish mortality from heart disease. Blood thinning herbs include **alfalfa** (*Medicago sativa*), **birch** (*Betula*), **sweet clover** (*Melilotus*), **bedstraws** (*Galium*), **poplar** (*Populus*), **red clover** (*Trifolium pratense*), **willow** (*Salix*), and **wintergreen** (*Gaultheria procumbens*). A daily spoonful of a vinegar made from the leaves, buds, and/or flowers of any of these provides the benefits of aspirin and some extras: minerals to keep your bones in top shape and acid to improve digestion.

### Step 5a. Use supplements . . .

★ Women who take **vitamin E** supplements during and after menopause have a 36 percent lower risk of heart attack. A recent WHO study concluded that a low level of vitamin E in the blood was the most important predictor of death from heart disease.

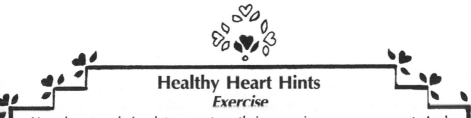

## Healthy Heart Hints
### Exercise

Your heart and circulatory system thrive on vigorous movement. And frequent small doses of physical activity are more heart healthy than infrequent heavy workouts. Thirty minutes of exercise a day will do, and you can do it in little pieces. **Nettle** infusion increases stamina and energy. A cup for breakfast and another at lunch will make you *want* to exercise, you'll be so full of get-up-and-go.

◇ For every hour you work take a five-minute break; stretch and walk.
◇ Use your five minute break to climb up five flights of stairs (you can take the elevator down).
◇ Keep a jump rope or a frisky dog handy.
◇ Work in one room and keep all your supplies in another so you have to get up over and over to fetch things.
◇ Turn on dance music while you wash dishes and sweep up.
◇ Go on a camping trip at least once this year.
◇ Become friends with someone who loves to exercise.

★ **Niacin** supplements reduce mortality from heart problems as well as estrogen when used for 7-10 years. Niacin does not promote cancer, is fairly inexpensive, and is available without prescription.

Recommended dose of niacin (*not niacinamide*) is 500 mg with meals (three times a day). CAUTION: Initially, niacin causes a hot-flash-like flush for about 30 minutes after you ingest it. The more regularly you take it, the less often you will flush, if at all. Discontinue if you become nauseated or experience any gastrointestinal distress. Do not take niacin supplements if you have gout, diabetes, liver disease, gastric ulcers, or coronary heart disease. Avoid time-release capsules.

### Step 5b. Use drugs . . .

• Cardiovascular disease in post-menopausal women was reduced 32 percent in women who took 1-6 aspirins a week, as opposed to women who took no aspirin. Be aware, however, that daily use of aspirin can contribute to cerebral hemorrhage and gastrointestinal disorders, including bleeding ulcers.

• ERT, taken for 5-10 years, may reduce risk of cardiovascular diseases.

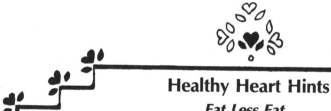

## Healthy Heart Hints
### Eat Less Fat

There is little argument about the benefit of a low-fat diet for the post-menopausal woman. High-fat diets encourage breast and colon cancers as well as cardiovascular disease (three top killers of crones).

◊ Eat meat once a week or less.

◊ Use only olive oil (low-heat cooking) and flax seed oil (at the table). If you must cheat a little, make it real butter, never margarine.

◊ Throw a soy drink (in a foil bag, not a box, which may burst when it freezes) in the freezer and eat it when you long for ice cream.

◊ Do enjoy your eggs, they're full of heart healthy lecithin; don't worry about the cholesterol. I prefer eggs produced by free-range chickens.

◊ Buy some crunchy kelp from Ryan Drum (see page 182) and snack on that instead of chips.

# Osteoporosis

*"Metamorphosis means complete Change, great granddaughter," says Grandmother Growth, in time to her drum beat. (Or is that your heart?) "And menopause is metamorphosis. To change completely, you must dissolve the old outline, then fill in the new one. As a baby Crone, you saw your rigidity soften, your will power dissolve, your very bones growing open. Now you are ready to reform yourself, to recast yourself, to create a new standing for yourself in your community."*

### Step 1. Collect information . . .

There is a certain chill slide of fear in thinking about osteoporosis: the fearful sound of bone breaking as you bend over to pick up a book, the fear of being a stooped old lady, the fear of an accidental slip that breaks a hip, landing you in the wheelchair, or even the grave. (As many as 30 percent of those over sixty who break a hip in North America will die as a direct result.)

Osteoporosis (loss of bone mass) and broken bones are deeply, but incorrectly, linked in our minds. Osteoporosis means the bones are thinner, not necessarily more prone to breakage. In a study of women aged sixty and older, low bone mass *did not* correlate with higher rates of fracture. In other words, osteoporosis does not always equal broken bones.

Nor is good bone mass reliable insurance against breakage. The American College of Physicians says: "The majority of women with hip fracture have a density of the hip that is within the normal range."

If keeping my bone mass up won't prevent fractures, what will?

*"Dear daughter," chuckles Grandmother Growth, "the answer is simple, though it may surprise you: chop wood, carry water, grow and eat your own organic vegetables (and the weeds), and take time to enjoy yourself."*

It is unclear whether, or how much, calcium or ERT can lower fracture rates. (See box.) But exercise does lower fracture rates. Those whose daily lives include some strenuous activities have the fewest post-menopausal fractures; those whose daily lives are the least active have the greatest incidence of post-menopausal fractures.

In areas of the world where women live long and maintain strong bones, daily life includes long walks carrying water and/or firewood. Many of these women eat far, far less calcium than we are told we need, and none of them take hormones after menopause, yet broken hips and "dowager's hump" are virtually unknown among them.

## Osteoporosis Risk Factors

*You are a woman at a high risk of osteoporosis-related fractures if you say "yes" to four or more of these statements:*

◇ I am white-skinned with a fair complexion.
◇ I am thin/petite.
◇ I smoke cigarettes every day.
◇ I have at least 10 alcoholic drinks (including beers, wine coolers) per week.
◇ I drink at least three cups of coffee a day.
◇ I eat animal protein at least twice a day.
◇ I eat salty, processed food regularly (chips, canned goods, lunch meats).
◇ I drink soda (even "healthy" kinds) daily.
◇ My ovaries were removed (or ceased functioning) before I turned 40.
◇ I breast-fed two or more children before the age of 25.
◇ I have given birth to more than six children.
◇ I have never been pregnant.
◇ I frequently diet or fast; was/am anorexic/bulimic.
◇ I was malnourished as a child or as a teenager.
◇ I have a family history of osteoporosis.
◇ I work sitting down/am restricted to wheelchair or bed/ don't exercise.
◇ At times I have exercised to the point where I lost my period.
◇ I am lactose intolerant/have not eaten dairy for ten years.
◇ I did/do receive long-term adrenal steroid/cortisone therapy.
◇ I take diuretics on a regular basis.
◇ I take anticonvulsants such as Dilantin or phenobarbitol.
◇ I have kidney disease/am on dialysis.
◇ I have chronic diarrhea/often take antacids/am a gastrectomy patient.
◇ I am hyperthyroid/parathyroid/take thyroid medication.
◇ I am diabetic.

**NOTE:** *High-risk women will benefit from exercise and organically grown foods, even if, especially if, they elect to use estrogen or calcium supplements.*

I chop some wood and I carry some water; I grow my own vegetables and weeds; and I do celebrate joyously. If you can't or don't, here are some other ways to build (and mend) your crone bones.

Note: For three to seven years post-menopausally, the following remedies and preventions for osteoporosis shouldn't be expected to produce very noticeable results. They may be worth using, however, so you'll be in the habit of exercising and eating calcium-rich foods. As an older crone, you can use these remedies to *reverse* osteoporosis; once the menopausal **Change** is complete, bone mass is easily rebuilt with Wise Woman ways.

### Step 2. Engage the energy . . .

• **Safety first.** Preventable falls are the biggest cause of broken bones, especially after the age of seventy, when 90 percent of all hip fractures occur. What to do? Install safety bars in your bathroom. Test vision and hearing regularly. Adopt sensible shoes. Make carrying a cane fashionable. Beware the effects of alcohol and prescription drugs.

★ Natural vitamin D is critical for flexible, strong bones. It is made by your skin in the presence of **sunlight**. Post-menopausal women with severe bone deterioration usually lack adequate amounts of vitamin D in their blood. Even 5-10 minutes of sunlight daily will do it.

★ If you have early warning signs of weakening bones (see box), try this **visualization** once or twice a day for at least three weeks. Stand in front of a mirror. Pretend that you can see through your skin and muscles. See yourself as a skeleton. See your bones as very white, chalky white, thick milky white, dense cooked-egg white, blank piece of paper white, thick, white, dense, white.

• The homeopathic cell salt *Silica* is recommended for those at risk of severe osteoporosis.

### Step 3. Nourish and tonify . . .

• **Exercise** and a **calcium-rich diet** reversed osteoporosis in a year-long study of 36 post-menopausal women. Bone mass in the spine increased by 0.5 percent in those who exercised (a vigorous 50 minute walk four times a week), irrespective of calcium levels (non-exercisers lost 7 percent of spine bone mass that year). Thigh bone density increased by 2 percent in those getting generous amounts of calcium (1650 mg daily from food and supplements) and decreased by 1.1 percent in the low-calcium group (under 1000 mg daily). (Miriam Nelson, et al., Tufts/ American Journal of Clinical Nutrition, May 1991.)

★ Leg lifts and arm lifts with **weights** improve your balance, increase

## Early Signs of Osteoporosis

◇ Persistent backache, especially in the lower back.
◇ Severe or sudden periodontal disease, gum infections, loose teeth.
◇ Sudden insomnia and restlessness.
◇ Nightly leg and foot cramps.
◇ Gradual loss of height. Check yearly by measuring from fingertip to fingertip (arms outstretched) then down your back from head to heels. The measurements should be equal.

## Calcium & ERT & Broken Bones

The correlations between ERT/HRT, calcium supplementation, and the actual *incidence of fracture* are not clear, though it is well established that both ERT and a calcium-rich diet can halt or reverse osteoporosis once the immediate post-menopausal period is over.

**ERT** slows osteoporosis by slowing bone cell death. It does not nourish bone cell growth, however, so there is still some bone loss. In fact, bone loss occurs quite rapidly in women who take ERT for a while and then stop. The risk of fracture is estimated to decrease by as much as 40-60 percent for the woman who takes estrogen for at least ten years.

**Calcium** builds bone mass, but doesn't affect the rate of bone cell death. Foods or supplements equalling 1500 mg daily are recommended for post-menopausal women. With this intake, the risk of fracture is said to be reduced by 50-75 percent. Yet the countries with the highest incidence of osteoporosis-related fractures are the very countries whose citizens consume the most calcium! (They also consume the most protein, and are the least physically fit.)

bone strength, and help maintain flexibility. Begin with 1 pound/.5 kilo weights and increase gradually to 4-5 pounds/2 kilos on each side. Sit in a sturdy hard-backed chair (wheelchair is fine), or lie down on your back in bed. Lift one foot or hand until the limb is straight out in front of you. Hold for 1-3 seconds; lower and rest for 1-3 seconds. Repeat no more than 10 times on each side for each arm and leg.

*"My grandmother started doing these weighted lifts last year when she turned 100. This year, at 101, she fell backwards over a planter and landed hard on her hips, suffering no more than a bruise and some loss of dignity."*

★ **Horsetail** (*Equisetum arvense*) is my favorite herb for restoring bone density. Through its synergistic mineral actions, it helps the bone thicken and stabilize. A daily tea of the dried, spring-picked herb helps reverse osteoporosis and speeds healing of fractures. An average-sized woman in her 60s successfully healed three broken vertebrae (from a skiing accident) with horsetail/comfrey leaf infusion and was back on the slopes, cautiously, in less than three months.

• Older stomachs may not produce enough hydrochloric acid to free calcium and other minerals and allow them to be absorbed into the tissues. **Dandelion** root tincture, 10-15 drops taken before meals, will remedy this.

★ Review information on **calcium** in "Preventing Osteoporosis." Include in your daily diet at least three of the following:
  ☞ 1 teaspoon/5 ml seaweed such as kelp or wakami
  ☞ 2 cups/500 ml fresh or 1 cup/250 ml cooked dark greens
  ☞ 1 cup/250 ml of yogurt or whey
  ☞ a big mug/300 ml of calcium-rich herbal infusion (see page 190)
  ☞ 1 tablespoon/15 ml herbal vinegar (see page 192)
  ☞ 1 tablespoon/15 ml lemon juice in which egg shell has soaked overnight
  ☞ 2 tablespoons/30 ml blackstrap molasses

★ **Micronutrients** such as selenium, chromium, copper, boron, silicon, zinc, cobalt, and sulfur are vital for flexible strength in bones. Richest sources are common weeds (including seaweeds, nettles, dandelion) and organically grown grains and produce.

*"Osteoporosis can be induced by a diet deficient in any of about ten micronutrients."*     –From a study on dietary causes of osteoporosis

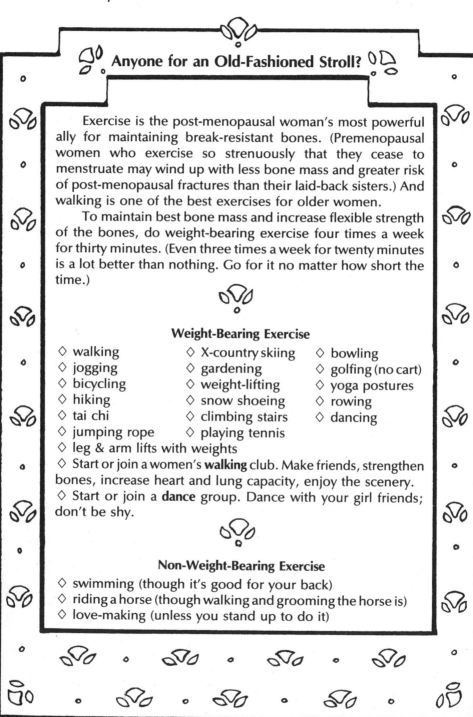

## Anyone for an Old-Fashioned Stroll?

Exercise is the post-menopausal woman's most powerful ally for maintaining break-resistant bones. (Premenopausal women who exercise so strenuously that they cease to menstruate may wind up with less bone mass and greater risk of post-menopausal fractures than their laid-back sisters.) And walking is one of the best exercises for older women.

To maintain best bone mass and increase flexible strength of the bones, do weight-bearing exercise four times a week for thirty minutes. (Even three times a week for twenty minutes is a lot better than nothing. Go for it no matter how short the time.)

### Weight-Bearing Exercise

◇ walking                ◇ X-country skiing      ◇ bowling
◇ jogging                ◇ gardening             ◇ golfing (no cart)
◇ bicycling              ◇ weight-lifting        ◇ yoga postures
◇ hiking                 ◇ snow shoeing          ◇ rowing
◇ tai chi                ◇ climbing stairs       ◇ dancing
◇ jumping rope           ◇ playing tennis
◇ leg & arm lifts with weights
◇ Start or join a women's **walking** club. Make friends, strengthen bones, increase heart and lung capacity, enjoy the scenery.
◇ Start or join a **dance** group. Dance with your girl friends; don't be shy.

### Non-Weight-Bearing Exercise

◇ swimming (though it's good for your back)
◇ riding a horse (though walking and grooming the horse is)
◇ love-making (unless you stand up to do it)

### Step 4. Stimulate/Sedate . . .

• Those who drink 2-3 cups of coffee daily, whether regular or decaffeinated, increase their risk of osteoporosis-related fractures by 69 percent; those who drink more than 3 cups a day increase their risk by 82 percent. (American Journal of Epidemiology, Oct. 1990.)

*"Osteoporosis-related fractures are easy to prevent: just decrease coffee and alcohol, increase exercise and calcium."*        –New York City gynecologist

• **Weak electrical charges** are sometimes machine-generated to stimulate bone growth. You can stimulate weak electrical charges yourself to help increase your bone mass or heal fractures. Try:
  ☞ massage
  ☞ weight-bearing exercise (see box)
  ☞ sexual tension and release
  ☞ hands-on energy treatments
  ☞ herbal poultices
  ☞ isometric exercise
  ☞ prayer and imagination
  ☞ pressing with fingertips into the middle undersides of both feet
  ☞ acupuncture
  ☞ magnets

### Step 5a. Use supplements . . .

★ **Wild yam cream**, available through Pro-Tec (800-648-8211), contains a naturally derived progesterone. Progesterone increases the rate of bone formation and remodeling. Studies have shown a diminution of bone loss in post-menopausal women using this cream.

*"The signs and symptoms of osteoporosis cleared in every patient [using a progesterone cream] and the incidence of fractures dropped to zero."*
—JR Lee, MD, Lancet, Nov. 24, 1990

• Supplements of up to 50,000 units of **beta carotene** daily increase progesterone production and protect bones.

★ **Microcrystalline hydroxapatite** is specifically formulated to deposit minerals into the bones. Clinical practitioners say it consistently helps reverse osteoporosis and heal compression fractures in the spine.

★ **Vitamin D** supplements may be needed for those who cannot spend enough time in the sun. The recommended dose is high: 400-800 IU daily. In the elderly, vitamin D toxicity begins at 2000 IU per day.

• If boron-rich organic produce and grains are not part of your diet, you may wish to supplement with 3 mg **boron** daily.

- **Calcium supplements** are not nearly as effective as a calcium-rich diet. But if you do want to take a calcium supplement, see page 26. CAUTION: Women who took 75 mg of sodium fluoride and 1500 mg of calcium daily for four years had denser neck, back, and thigh bones, but significantly *more* arm, leg, wrist, rib, and hip *fractures* than a control group. (New England Journal of Medicine, 1990.)

- **Fluoride**, sometimes prescribed as a cure for osteoporosis, increases bone density but also increases osteoporosis-related fractures. Post-menopausal women drinking water containing 4 parts fluoride per million incur more than twice as many fractures as their counterparts whose drinking water has little or no fluoride (regardless of the amount of calcium ingested). (Mary Sowers, University of Michigan/American Journal of Epidemiology April, 1991.)

Fluoride is found not only in drinking water, but also in canned foods, soda pop, and residues from insecticides and fertilizers on produce. These "hidden" sources may constitute as much as half of your daily fluoride intake. Post-menopausal women may wish to question their dentists on the advisability of fluoride treatments and toothpastes.

### Step 5b. Use drugs . . .

- We are enjoined to take estrogen replacement pills (ERT) to "prevent osteoporosis." I think it's important to remember that some osteoporosis is an inevitable part of the menopausal **Change**. Virtually all women lose 5-10 percent of their bone mass in the five years after menopause.

For a post-menopausal woman to ask: "Osteoporosis, how can I prevent it?" is like asking "How can I prevent the sun from setting each evening?" When we try to prevent the natural flows of life, we begin to think that these natural processes (such as bone thinning with age and menopause itself) are problems, which we are told we need to "cure" by technological means. In the case of osteoporosis, computerized scans of bone density during and right after menopause lead almost inevitably to a prescription for estrogen therapy, the supposed cure for the natural process.

But even high-tech medicine can't forestall the **Change**: in one study, ERT, given to women just after their menses stopped, slowed bone loss for only 3-9 months. After that time, bone loss resumed, and at a much accelerated rate, even though ERT was continued.

★ **HRT** is probably the better choice of hormones to maintain bones, if that's the way you wish to go. Progesterone is as important to bones as estrogen. But the progestine or progestagen you'd be taking is synthetic, and the risks are not well established.

• A synthetic version of the parathyroid hormone calcitonin can be injected to slow bone breakdown if exercise, diet, and supplements are not sufficient to restore bone strength and flexibility.

• When vertebrae are breaking from compression and the bones seem to break at a touch, a diphosphonate named etidronate (Didronel) can stop bone cells from breaking down by coating them in a crystalline covering.

### Step 6. Break and enter . . .

• Bone density measurements are invasive diagnostic techniques, not preventive measures. They go hand in hand with hormone therapy. If you do not intend to take ERT, there is absolutely no reason for you to have your bone mass measured.

*"There are no studies of the effectiveness of early detection in achieving decreased incidence of fracture or of bone demineralization."*
                                    –The Canadian Task Force on Periodic Health Exams

• How come high-tech, high-cost bone density measurements are being promoted as essential screening procedures for all women over 40, even though only one-quarter of all white women, and far fewer women of color, will develop severe osteoporosis? In addition to being fairly expensive, bone mass tests are basically useless in helping predict osteoporosis-related fractures. As we have seen (step 1), the density of bone is not an accurate predictor of resistance to fracture. And the *rate* of bone loss cannot be estimated very well as it is neither constant nor predictable in any person.

## Mending Broken Bones

*"Knowing a woman's age is almost as good in predicting her risk of fracture as is measuring her bone mass."* –AMA, 1989

### Step 1. Collect information . . .

Obviously, it is preferable to prevent broken bones rather than heal them, but many women simply don't realize they have a problem until a minor fall breaks a wrist or ankle. Even during the immediate post-menopausal years, when bone loss is rapid, these remedies will help you heal broken bones more quickly and with fewer complications. They are wonderful allies for women undergoing total hip replacement as well.

If you wonder if you've broken a bone, but don't want to be X-rayed, try this. Place a vibrating tuning fork at one end of the bone in question. Then at the other end. If the bone is intact, the vibration will be pleasant; if broken, the vibration will be painful or uncomfortable.

In many instances, bones mend better in a splint rather than a cast. Ask your helper/doctor for a splint you can remove easily, so poultices and massages can be used to promote healing.

### Step 2. Engage the energy . . .

• Shine a **blue light** on the broken bone, or visualize blue light surrounding it. This can significantly reduce the pain.

• Hatha **yoga postures** help the mending bones and muscles stay strong and vital. Find an experienced teacher and ask for help.

★ Bones lay down new cells best when there is a weak **electrical charge** passing through the bone. (See page 161.) Even imagining that you are exercising the broken limb increases the electrical flow!

• Energy treatments of any kind, **reiki** or soft **polarity**, for instance, are very beneficial for mending bones.

• How is this a *break*through for you at the most basic/bone level?

### Step 3. Nourish and tonify . . .

★ **Horsetail** sparks strong new bone cell growth. Add a teaspoon/ 1 gram of the dried herb to a cup of boiling water, steep 5 minutes, and drink. Or add a tablespoon/3 grams of horsetail to an ounce/30 grams of any one of the following bone-mending herbs and infuse in 1 quart/ liter of boiling water. Try to drink the entire amount each day.

☞ nettle leaves          ☞ alfalfa
☞ comfrey leaves       ☞ sage leaves
☞ red clover blossoms    ☞ oatstraw with seed
☞ raspberry leaves      ☞ uva ursi leaves

• Insure infection-free healing and prevent nerve damage by using 25-30 drops of **St. Joan's wort** (*Hypericum*) tincture once or twice a day.

### Step 4. Sedate/Stimulate . . .

★ **Skullcap** tincture eases pain from broken bones and calms fears. Try 3-5 drops every 30 minutes until pain eases, then as needed. Large doses are quite sleep inducing, but never habit-forming, in my experience.

★ Stimulate repair of muscle, tendon, ligament, and bone cells with **comfrey** infusions and poultices. Pour boiling water over fresh or dried *Symphytum* leaves. While they steep, find a thin towel or soft cloth to lay over the injured limb. Place the very warm comfrey leaves on cloth and cover them with plastic wrap and a layer of towels. Remove when cool. Drink a cup or more of infusion daily.

(Steps 5a, 5b, and 6 omitted on purpose.)

Osteoporosis
# References & Resources

"Calcium supplementation of the diet," JA Kanis & R Passmore, British Medical Journal, Jan. 1989

"The Calcium Controversy: Finding a Middle Ground Between the Extremes," RP Heaney, MD, Public Health Reports, Oct. 1988

"Healthy Bones Year After Year," National Osteoporosis Foundation, Prevention, Nov. 1990

"Hormonal and Nutritional Aspects of Osteoporosis," JR Lee, MD, 1991

National Osteoporosis Foundation, 2100 M St. NW, Suite 602, Washington, DC 20037

"Osteoporosis," Science News, Vol. 138, No. 18, Nov. 1990

"Osteoporosis," MN Mead, *EastWest*, March 1990

"Osteoporosis: More Calcium is not the Answer," Karen & J. Ehmke, Ontario's Common Ground Magazine, Summer 1990

"Osteoporosis Screening: Pro and Con," Marianne Whatley & Meredith DuHamel, National Women's Health Network News, Feb. 1989

"Progesterone and the Prevention of Osteoporosis," J. Prior, MD, Y. Vigna, RN, N. Alojado, RN, Canadian Journal of Ob/Gyn, Vol. 3, No. 4, 1991

"Stone Age Bones," SB Eaton, MD, Longevity, March 1990

"Strong Bone Test: Should You Take It?" Robin Henig, Longevity, Apr. 1990

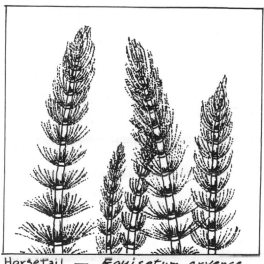

Horsetail — *Equisetum arvense*

# My Aching Joints

*"Keep moving, keep moving, bend and flow, bend and flow, sweet sister,"*
*the ever-so-faint whisper of Grandmother Growth's voice plays around*
*your ears. "Keep your wise blood circulating in your belly, moving*
*through your spine, and flowing into action. Stay loose, stretch, reach,*
*retain your flexibility. Move, flow, bend, and grow, sweet sister, grow."*

### Step 1. Collect information . . .

Whether it is age or changing hormones, more than half of all post-
menopausal women experience occasional to severe joint pain. (Twice
as many women as men suffer from aching joints.)

Aching knees, elbows, and shoulders are the most frequent aching
joints at menopause. Aching hips, lower back, wrist joints often indicate
deeper distresses such as worsening osteoporosis, kidney weakness,
or immune system dysfunction.

Don't ignore aching, swollen joints. Osteoarthritis (stiff, achy, lumpy,
swollen, hot, noisy joints) can degenerate the joints. Rheumatoid arthritis (swollen, tender joints, sometimes accompanied by fever or fatigue)
is an auto-immune disorder that can progressively deform joints until
function is lost. But early treatment, especially when the joint begins
to ache, can effect a cure and forestall further occurrences of arthritis.

### Step 2. Engage the energy . . .

★ **Visualization** for women with aching joints: Sit or lie in a posture
that is comfortable for you and imagine that your aching joints are
getting hotter and hotter. When they are as hot as you can bear,
imagine the joints getting colder and colder. Go back and forth at least
four times, ending at a temperature that feels just right.

• To help aching hips, shoulders, knees, elbows, find a **hatha yoga**
teacher and attend class regularly. Joint mobility increases rapidly with
the focused attention and gentle stretching of yoga postures.

• The majority of post-menopausal women who exposed their painful
joints to light shining through a blue filter for 15 minutes a day experienced significant pain relief from their rheumatoid arthritis.

• Homeopathic *Hypericum* is the general remedy for sore joints.

**Step 3. Nourish and tonify . . .**

★ **White birch**, Weissbirke, Boleau blanc (*Betula alba* and most other *Betula* species) is a recommended remedy for the post-menopausal woman with arthritis, uric acid build-up in the joints (gout), calcium spurs in the heels and feet, heart/kidney edema, arteriosclerosis, high cholesterol, hypertension, obesity, and chronic cystitis. A dose of the tincture of fresh leaves or leaf buds is 1-2 dropperfuls (25-50 drops) up to three times a day; of the tea of the dried leaves, as much as you like.

★ **Black currant** bud macerate is anti-inflammatory (soothing to aching joints) and hormone-helping (strengthening to bones). And a wonderful ally for the post-menopausal woman with arthritis, rheumatism, allergies, headaches, and persistent hot flashes. Use a 30-50 drop dose up to three times a day.

• **Swimming in warm water** is one of the safest ways to exercise joints, no matter what's causing the ache.

★ **Moxibustion** is one of my favorite tonifying techniques for sore joints. The smoky warmth of the burning *Artemisia* eases pain and keeps joints open and flexible.

★ Massage **arnica** or **St. Joan's wort** oil into the painful joint for amazing relief. Or apply a fresh **chickweed poultice**.

• Essential fatty acids are anti-inflammatory. Get them from fresh flax seed or evening primrose oil. A spoonful several times a day often relieves pain within a few days. Regular use helps prevent aching joints.

**Step 4. Sedate/Stimulate . . .**

• Cold vegetables on hot joints are a great blessing. Try a poultice of tofu, grated raw potato, or squash.

★ **Acupuncture** treatments are quite effective in relieving chronic joint pain. A more "modern" equivalent is trans-cutaneous electrical nerve stimulation (TENS).

★ **Ginger** baths, soaks, and compresses bring soothing, warm relief to sore and aching joints.

★ Sweat lodges, saunas, steam baths, mud baths, and mineral soaks penetrate the joints with intense heat and initiate healing energy and movement in the area.

★ Some women report dramatic improvement in joint mobility and lack of pain when they eliminate one or all of these foods from their regular diet: sugar, nightshades (potatoes, tomatoes, eggplant, peppers), citrus, dairy products, meat, vegetable oils (excluding olive oil), MSG, alcohol.

• **Poke** (*Phytolacca americana* and other species) and **devil's club** (*Oplopanax*) are unusual plants of the east and west coasts of North America, respectively. The roots of both have long-lived reputations for easing joint pains, especially from rheumatoid arthritis. Dose of either root tinctured (do not used dried poke root) is 1-4 drops daily. Poke berries may be taken as well: 1-2 dried whole berries each morning. (The toxic seeds pass harmlessly through the digestive tract if you swallow the berries without chewing.) CAUTION: Poke root and poke berry seeds are considered highly toxic. I have used the low doses recommended here for more than fifteen years with highly favorable results.

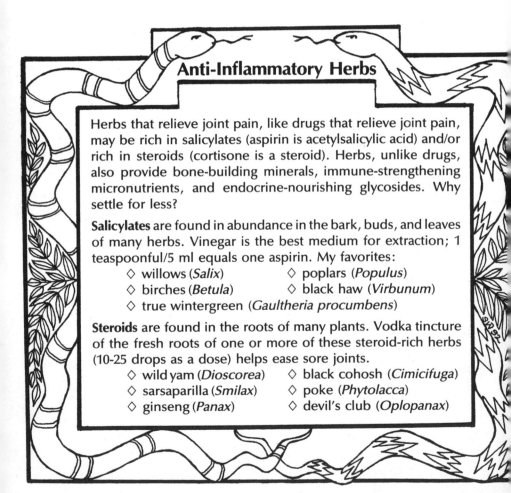

## Anti-Inflammatory Herbs

Herbs that relieve joint pain, like drugs that relieve joint pain, may be rich in salicylates (aspirin is acetylsalicylic acid) and/or rich in steroids (cortisone is a steroid). Herbs, unlike drugs, also provide bone-building minerals, immune-strengthening micronutrients, and endocrine-nourishing glycosides. Why settle for less?

**Salicylates** are found in abundance in the bark, buds, and leaves of many herbs. Vinegar is the best medium for extraction; 1 teaspoonful/5 ml equals one aspirin. My favorites:

- ◇ willows (*Salix*)
- ◇ birches (*Betula*)
- ◇ true wintergreen (*Gaultheria procumbens*)
- ◇ poplars (*Populus*)
- ◇ black haw (*Virbunum*)

**Steroids** are found in the roots of many plants. Vodka tincture of the fresh roots of one or more of these steroid-rich herbs (10-25 drops as a dose) helps ease sore joints.

- ◇ wild yam (*Dioscorea*)
- ◇ sarsaparilla (*Smilax*)
- ◇ ginseng (*Panax*)
- ◇ black cohosh (*Cimicifuga*)
- ◇ poke (*Phytolacca*)
- ◇ devil's club (*Oplopanax*)

**Step 5b. Use drugs . . .**

• Literally tons of non-steroidal anti-inflammatory drugs (NSAIDs), such as aspirin and ibuprofen, are sold yearly in North America. (See anti-inflammatory herbs: salicylates.)

• Steroidal drugs are frequently used to ease chronic joint pain. Unfortunate side effects include stimulation of osteoporosis and suppression of the immune system. Steroid-rich herbs don't produce these side effects. (See anti-inflammatory herbs: steroids.)

**Step 6. Break and enter . . .**

• Injection of cortisone into the affected joint may sometimes offer prompt relief. The trade-off is the deep harm done to your immune system. And sometimes it doesn't work at all.

• Ditto for gold injections.

# Foot and Leg Cramps, Numbness

**Step 1. Collect information . . .**

Frequent leg and foot cramps or numbness of the extremities may be an annoying minor problem during or after menopause, or a symptom of some deeper distress. (See box.) The two most common causes of night cramps in post-menopausal women are use of tobacco and inactivity of the legs. These remedies helped our grannies get around.

**Step 2. Engage the energy . . .**

• Try a warm **foot bath** with a few drops of essential oil of **peppermint** or **rosemary** right before bed.

**Step 3. Nourish and tonify . . .**

★ Ingest more **calcium**-rich foods. (See page 25.)

★ **Black haw** tincture or tincture of **St. Joan's wort** blossoms helps prevent and relieve muscle cramps. Try 20-25 drops just before bed. Keep it handy for quick relief when cramps wake you at night.

• If your legs twitch and move and keep you awake all night (restless leg syndrome), you are probably anemic. Remedy with 10-20 drops of **yellow dock** root tincture daily.

### Step 4. Sedate/Stimulate . . .

• A **hot bath** right before bed soothes muscles, increases blood flow, and can help get you smoothly through the night. Add **valerian** to the bath to promote deep sleep.

★ "As a pubescent girl, I had terrible foot cramps that would bring me bolt upright out of my sleep. I learned to keep a glass cola bottle under my bed. I got relief in seconds by pressing and rolling the bottle hard along the floor with my foot."

### Step 5a. Use supplements . . .

• A **calcium/magnesium** supplement (500 mg) taken at bedtime often relieves foot and leg cramps during the night.

• If that doesn't do it, add a 100 mg niacin supplement.

• Vitamin E supplements also help relieve cramping of the legs at night. See page 62 for doses and cautions.

• Numbness and cramping of the legs can be symptoms of an overdose or depletion of vitamin $B_6$.

### Step 5b. Use drugs . . .

• Antidepressant drugs can cause writhing and aching sensations deep in the legs.

• Quinine is an old standby that still helps wonderfully well.

---

## Numb/Cramped Feet and Legs

Your frequently numb legs and cramped calves and feet could be caused by:

◊ Heart problems; use cardiotonic herbs, see pages 151-3.
◊ Osteoporosis; see pages 155-163.
◊ Smoking tobacco; hints for stopping on page 150.
◊ Inactivity; five-minute exercises on page 153.
◊ Hypothyroidism (low thyroid activity). Take your waking temperature for several mornings; if it is consistently below 97.8°F, suspect hypothyroidism. Use seaweed to increase available iodine. Inquire about supplementation with thyroid hormones. Note that alcohol, coffee, tobacco, and white sugar depress thyroid function.

# References & Resources
## Chapter 3: Post-Menopause

"The Crone," Barbara Walker, Harper, 1986

"Grandmother of Time," Z Budapest, Harper & Row, 1989

"Growing Older, Getting Better: A Handbook for the Second Half of Life," Jane Porcino, Addison Wesley, 1983

HealthFacts, Center for Medical Consumers, 237 Thompson St., NY, NY 10012 • $21 for 12 sensible, readable newsletters.

"Johns Hopkins Medical Letter on Health After 50," 550 North Broadway, Suite 1100, Baltimore, MD 21205

"Look Me in the Eye: Old Women, Aging and Ageism," Barbara Macdonald, Spinsters/Aunt Lute, 1983

"Natural Health, Natural Medicine," A. Weil, MD, Houghton Mifflin, 1990

"No Stone Unturned: The Life and Times of Maggie Kuhn," Christina Long & Laura Quinn, Ballantine, 1991

"Ourselves, Growing Older," Paula Doress, Simon & Schuster, 1990

"Peace Pilgrim," Herself, Ocean Tree, 1982

"Risks, Benefits of Estrogen Use Remain Unclear," JE Bishop, Wall Street Journal, Nov. 1991

"Shakti Woman," Vicki Noble, Harper, 1991

"Taking Hormones and Women's Health: Choices, Risks, Benefits," National Women's Health Network, 1989

"What Are You Doing with the Rest of Your Life," Paula Payne Hardin, New World Library, 1992

"When I am an Old Woman I Shall Wear Purple," Sandra Martz (ed.), Papier Mache, 1990

"Women and Aging: An Anthology," Calyx, ed., Calyx, 1990

"Women and the Crisis in Sex Hormones," Barbara & G. Seaman, Bantam, 1978

Insure a happy cronehood for yourself and others; consider joining:

• Gray Panthers, 1424 16th St NW, Suite 602, Washington DC 20036
• Older Women's League, 730 11th St NW, Suite 300, Wash., DC 20001
• Women's Initiative of AARP, 601 E St NW, Washington, DC 20049

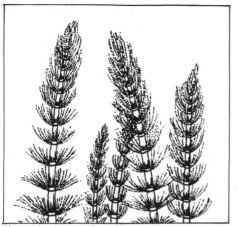

Horsetail — *Equisetum arvense*

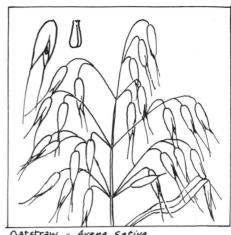

Oatstraw - *Avena Sativa*

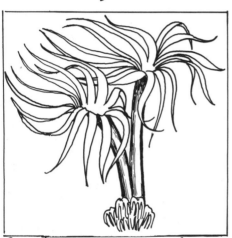

Sea palm — *Postelsia palmæformis*

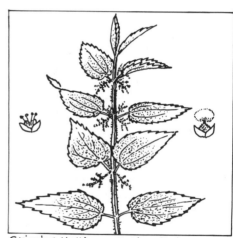

Stinging Nettle - *Urtica dioica*

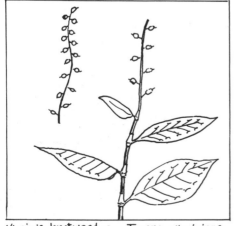

Virginia knotweed — *Tovara virginiana*

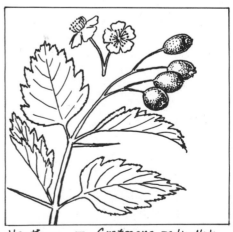

Hawthorn — *Cratægus pedicellata*

# Herbal Allies for Post-Menopausal Women

My favorite herbs for post-menopausal women are horsetail, oat-straw, stinging nettle, seaweeds, and the plants rich in flavonoids. These gentle green allies are more like foods than drugs; they offer bone-creating, heart-protecting, disease-preventing, sex-enhancing optimum nutrition to the woman in the second half of her life.

## Horsetail
### *Equisetum arvense*
Ackerschachtelhalm, Prêle des champs

Horsetail is particularly rich in silica and glycosides (which nourish hormones, heart, and bones), and is thus uniquely suited to be one of the post-menopausal woman's favorite allies.

Use spring-picked horsetail herb to:

• *Reverse osteoporosis*
• *Stimulate fracture-mending and bone repair*
Mineral-rich horsetail feeds the bones. Fractures and thin bones, no matter how old, mend and thicken rapidly with horsetail's help.

• *Stabilize and reverse gum disease and loss of jaw bone*
When there is good dental hygiene, but recurrent or chronic periodontal disease, a daily cup of horsetail tea often works wonderfully as a strong catalyst to restore health to the gums and replace bone lost from the jaw.

• *Relieve cystitis*
Horsetail has been recommended since the sixteenth century for all irritated conditions of the bladder and urinary tract. Note that plants harvested too late (more than 6-7 weeks of growth) may aggravate rather than soothe.

• *Reduce bloat*
• *Check menstrual hemorrhage*
• *Prevent clogged arteries, strengthen veins*
• *Ease persistent hot flashes*
Horsetail does all this by virtue of its abundant silica, chromium, flavonoids, saponins, and astringent agents. For even better effect, combine with stinging nettles.

• *Increase energy, reduce fatigue*
Horsetail supplies peppy potassium, merry magnesium, and strong-as-nails iron for building Crone power.

• *Nourish strong, healthy hair and fingernails*
Drinking horsetail does what you always hoped drinking gelatin would do: makes those nails strong and even. There are several commercial shampoos containing horsetail. Use some leftover infusion as a final rinse after you've washed your hair (if it's combined with nettle, all the better).

Horsetail herb is dictinctive and unusual in shape. I use it fresh for a soup "green" and dried for teas. *To avoid excess silica, and poisoning symptoms, pick horsetail in the spring only, for no more than a month after it emerges.* The tincture is ineffective in my experience; a vinegar might work. Add a big pinch of horsetail herb to any other herbal infusion, or enjoy as a simple. (See Bonny Bony Brew, Appendix 2)

**Dosage:** 1 cup/250 ml of tea of dried spring-gathered herb daily.
DO NOT USE if you experience sensations of nervous sensitivity or urinary irritability after consumption.

## Oatstraw Fan Club

★ Angela continued her pattern of premenstrual upset into her menopause, and was dubious that drinking the pleasant-tasting, mellow brew of oatstraw could have any effect on her "killing rage." Angela combined her oatstraw with a weekly yoga class and discovered she really wanted to paint. Two years later, she had her first piece in a show. "Rage is so much more interesting splashed across canvas," she told me, raising her cup of oatstraw with a wink.

*"After three weeks of drinking oatstraw infusion I realized that I felt more emotionally resilient, more capable in stressful situations, more on-center than I thought was possible."*

★ Vaginal dryness bothered Anne, but she was even more concerned that she seemed to have "misplaced my libido." Anne bought a big bag of sweet-smelling green oatstraw, drank her infusion morning and night, and did a sitz bath once a week. "Makes me too mellow to complain," she noted after the first week. Six weeks later, she called to say she felt sexier than she ever had, with plenty of lubrication. "Maybe it was the oatstraw," she mused, "and maybe I just needed to slow down and catch up with myself."

# Oatstraw
## *Avena sativa*
### Gruen Hafer, Avoine cultivée

Yes, the very same oats that you eat for breakfast are a special ally to women who wish they wouldn't "fly off the handle" so easily, to women who want to be sexy old ladies, and to women who treasure their bones. If you prefer, you may drink your oats instead of eating them. Or try *Avena* flower essence, recommended for the woman needing clarity about her life's direction. If you ally yourself with *Avena* expect her to help you:

- *Build strong, pliable bones*
- *Maintain firm, reliable teeth*

Rich in calcium — and the synergistic minerals and vitamins needed for best use of calcium — oatstraw has a well-deserved reputation for building tough, hardy folks with tough, hardy bones.

- *Stabilize blood sugar levels*
- *Relieve depression and emotional uproar*

Avena's steroidal saponins nourish the pancreas, liver, and adrenals and help prevent erratic blood sugar levels from playing havoc with your emotions.

- *Reduce cholesterol and risk of heart disease*
- *Improve circulatory functioning*

Oats and oatstraw can make your blood vessels more elastic, more vital. How will you notice? Your hemorrhoids and varicose veins will shrink, your heart rate will slow, and disturbances in your heart rate (such as palpitations and tachycardia) will diminish or disappear.

- *Nourish strong nerves*
- *Help you engage high energy currents*

Oatstraw and oats, both superior sources of the vitamin B complex, are exceptionally capable of helping women under stress.

- *Reduce frequency and duration of headaches*
- *Maintain restful sleep patterns*
- *Ease bladder spasms, incontinence, uterine pain, vaginal dryness*

Oatstraw in your teacup and oatstraw in your bathtub (see Appendix 2) relieves physical pains, emotional pains, and energy disturbances, while nourishing and strengthening vaginal, bladder, and urethral tissues.

- *Be an outrageous sexy old lady*

**Dosage: 1 cup/250 ml or more of dried leaf, stalk, and grain infusion daily.**

# Seaweeds

• *Prevent and relieve osteoporosis*
Seaweeds contain lavish amounts of every mineral needed to create and maintain solid bone mass. Kelp is an exceptionally rich source.

• *Lower blood pressure and cholesterol*
• *Eliminate varicose veins and hemorrhoids*
• *Restore and increase cardiac efficiency*
Japanese research confirms the cardiotonic and hypotensive effects of seaweed.

• *Relieve incontinence, vaginal dryness, and persistent hot flashes*
• *Nourish the glandular and urinary systems*
Seaweeds are superb sources of the nutrients most needed by the endocrine, circulatory, and immune systems. Regular use of seaweed helps maintain adequate production of all hormones.

• *Increase immune functioning*
• *Increase stamina*
• *Minimize the effects of stress, chemicals, and radiation*
• *Lengthen life span*
Algin in seaweed binds to damaging compounds and escorts them harmlessly out of the body. Free radicals are also eliminated with the assistance of vitamins E, C, and A, found abundantly in seaweeds. Use seaweed daily to improve health when faced with air pollution, unknown chemicals in the food supply, and the thinning ozone layer. Include at least ½ ounce/15 grams of brown seaweed (such as kelp or wakame) in the daily diet when healing from chemotherapy, radiation, and surgery. Use freely for several days before and after mammograms to help prevent damage to the cells from the X-rays.

• *Improve digestion*
• *Restore sexual interest and enjoyment*
• *Ease sore joints*
• *Bring a glossy glow to hair and skin*
As befits denizens of the ocean deep, seaweeds are especially good at nourishing juices: digestive juices, joint juices, emotional juices, erotic juices. Seaweed helps them all flow.

**Dosage:** For best results, use seaweed daily as a condiment, and at least once a week as a vegetable. Try it in soups, beans, and stir-frys. Sprinkle it on potatoes, pasta, grains, eggs, salads, popcorn. There is no known overdose. CAUTION: Avoid if you are hyperthyroid.

# Stinging Nettle
## *Urtica dioica, Urtica urens*
### Brennessel, Ortie

A few post-menopausal women tell me stinging nettle is too nourishing, too energizing; they found themselves unexpectedly having a normal menstrual flow after regular use of nettle. The more usual effects of nettle will be to:

- *Nourish, strengthen, rebuild kidneys and adrenals*
- *Ease and eliminate cystitis, bloat, and incontinence*
- *Rehydrate dry vaginal tissues*

Nettle has a miraculous ability to heal and restore adrenal/kidney functioning. I know of several women who never went on dialysis (as doctors suggested) and one who even went off it — thanks to sister spinster stinging nettle. Think of what she can do for your kidneys and adrenals if they aren't on the verge of failure! Nourish your post-menopausal adrenals with nettles and they'll produce enough estrogen to keep you looking and feeling juicy.

- *Create strong, flexible bones*

Nettle infusions, vinegars, and soups are fantastic sources of calcium, magnesium, potassium, silicon, boron, and zinc: the strong bone sisters. Nettles are also a source of vitamin D, necessary for keeping bones flexible.

- *Stabilize blood sugar*

Rich in chromium, manganese, and other nutrients restorative to glandular functioning, nettles, I suspect, help prevent adult onset diabetes.

- *Reduce fatigue and exhaustion; improve stamina*

Nettles nourish your energy at the deepest possible levels with intense supplies of iron, chlorophyll, and copper.

- *Reduce and eliminate headaches*
- *Nourish and support the immune system*
- *Nourish and heal the digestive system*
- *Nourish and strengthen the nervous system*
- *Prevent cancer*

Nettles are an optimum source of the vitamins critically important for health: vitamin B complex (especially thiamine, riboflavin, and niacin), carotenes (vitamin A), and vitamin C (ascorbic acid and bioflavonoids).

- *Nourish and energize the endocrine glands*
- *Nourish and rejuvenate the cardiovascular system*
- *Normalize weight*

• *Ease and prevent sore joints*
• *Relieve constipation and reduce hemorrhoids*
• *Nourish supple skin and healthy hair*
Nettles' super supplies of vitamins, minerals, proteins, and micro-nutrients nourish every bit of you, encouraging optimal functioning in all aspects of your being.

Enjoy cooked nettle greens all spring, but be sure to harvest and dry enough for winter-time infusions, too. Pick nettles only before the flowers emerge. Fresh leaves left to steep in olive oil impart a rich taste and innumerable healing qualities to the oil. And it makes a lovely vinegar as well.
*Dosage:* **1 cup/250 ml or more of dried leaf infusion daily.**

# Bioflavonoids

Plants containing flavonoids (from the Latin, *flavus*, yellow) were originally valued as dye plants. Today we appreciate them for many other reasons. Recent research on bioflavonoids (naturally occurring flavonoids) reveals them to be *anti-inflammatory, antihepatotoxic, anti-tumor, antimicrobial, antiviral, antioxidant, antiallergic, antiulcer, anal-gesic,* and *strengthening to the entire circulatory system,* from capil-laries to heart.

Bioflavonoids have an estrogenic effect, scientifically established as 1/50,000th the activity of estrogen. And bioflavonoids are essential to your ability to absorb ascorbic acid (vitamin C). No wonder plants exceptionally rich in flavonoids are such important allies for the post-menopausal woman.

**Regular use of bioflavonoid-rich herbs helps:**

☞ restore vaginal lubrication        ☞ decrease or end hot flashes
☞ improve pelvic tone              ☞ improve liver activity
☞ strengthen the bladder           ☞ lower risk of stroke & heart attack
☞ reduce water build-up in tissues  ☞ reduce muscle cramping
☞ ease sore joints                 ☞ improve resistance to infection

★ The richest source of bioflavonoids is the **inner skin of citrus** fruits. "Peel Power" is a lovely way to start the day. (See Appendix 2.)

★ **Buckwheat** greens, Buckweizen, Sarrasin (*Fagopyrum esculentum*) are an exceptional source of bioflavonoids. Grow them at home, like alfalfa sprouts, or buy them dried and made into tablets. (Kasha, the grain of buckwheat, does not contain bioflavonoids.) The wild equivalent is the leaves of **yellow dock** (*Rumex crispus*) or any knotweed (*Polygonum*).

★ **Elder**, Holunder, Sureau (*Sambucus nigra* and other species) is rich in bioflavonoids. I use the berries in jelly or wine, and the flowers for tinctures, wines, and salads.

★ **Hawthorn**, Weissdorn, Aubépine (*Crataegus oxycantha* and other species) offers berries, flowers, and leaves full of bioflavonoids. I use the berries to make jellies, wines, and a heart-strengthening tincture. The flowers and leaves, dried, make a wonderful tea.

★ **Horsetail**, Ackerschachtelhalm, Prêle des champs (*Equisetum arvense*) is best picked in the spring. I use it fresh in soups (not salads) and dried as a tea. (See page 173.)

• **Knotweeds**, Vogelknöterich, Renouée des oiseaux, Ho Shou Wu, (*Polygonaceae*) are well known for their abundance of bioflavonoids. In addition to buckwheat and yellow dock leaves, try the greens of any other knotweed local to your area.

• **Roses**, Hagrose, Rosier (*Rosa canina* and other species) are sisters to hawthorn and similarly abundant in bioflavonoids. I use fresh rose hips in jellies and wines and dry them for winter teas and soups. We eat the blossoms in salads and use glycerin to draw out the healing qualities of flower and leaf buds.

★ **Shepherd's purse**, Hirtentäschel, Capselle (*Capsella bursa-pastoris*) leaves are wonderful in salads. When it flowers, I use the whole fresh plant to make vinegar and vodka tinctures, capturing bioflavonoids for later use. (A dose is 25-50 drops three times daily.)

• **Sea buckthorn**, Sanddorn, Argousier (*Hippophae rhamnoides*) leaves are rich in many nutrients needed by post-menopausal women: bioflavonoids, carotenes (vitamin A), vitamin C, vitamin E, and the B vitamin complex, especially $B_6$. If you live where it grows, try it in salads.

• **Toadflax**, Frauenflachs, Linaire commune (*Linaria vulgaris*) flowers add flavonoids to salads. They can also be tinctured. (A dose is 15-20 drops.)

• **White dead nettle**, Weisse Taubnessel, Lamier blanc (*Lamium album*) doesn't sting, so try it in salads. Or dry bunches when it's flowering and get your flavonoids from the infusion.

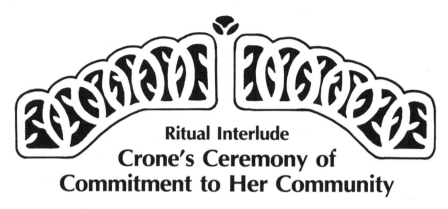

### Ritual Interlude
# Crone's Ceremony of Commitment to Her Community

As the menopausal years draw to a close and you find yourself more stable in your new self, feeling more like your "old self" as you become your older self, it is time to manifest the last stage of initiation: rebirth.

You've spent time in some form of isolation as you journeyed the unpredictable years of menopause. You have given death to your image of yourself as Mother and crowned yourself Crone. Now comes the time to reenter your community in your new role.

You return as Crone. You hold your wise blood inside. You have learned how to spiral the updrafts of hot flashes. You have learned detachment in the midst of emotional hurricanes. You have submitted yourself to chaos and have witnessed the most ancient of all mysteries. How can you share this with your community?

In the ancient past, in the days of the matriarchy, and in some matrifocal cultures yet, the woman who had completed her menopausal metamorphosis initiated young men into the ways of love play most pleasing to women. She was honored as the teller of truth and the keeper of peace. She was the keeper of traditions and the link to the spirit world.

Today, there are no givens, and we are each free to choose our own role as Crone. A ritual of commitment helps others know what your new role in your family and community will be. Here is one example to guide you.

\*   \*   \*   \*   \*

For this ritual, gather an audience of friends, family, and significant others, the more the better. You could compare it, at least in mood, to a wedding or a christening. Wait until at least thirteen moons after your Crone's Crowning ceremony.

Let there be music and sweet scents as you all gather. At the appointed time, call everyone to join hands. You alone remain outside the circle.

When the circle is complete, begin a hum, vibrating from the feet. Let it move and spiral until all are woven in and the group energy feels whole. With the hum of the group supporting you, ask light, breath, and inspiration, the powers of the east, to be present. Ask warmth, nourishment, and protection, the powers of the south, to be present. Ask emotion, fluidity, and compassion, the powers of the west, to be present. Ask stillness, patience, wisdom, the powers of the north, to be present. Ask the above and the below to be present. Ask the inner core of each person to be present.

Ask the circle to open and include you, symbolizing your return to community life. In your own words affirm: "I stand before you as self-initiated Crone, woman of wholeness. Though I have lived for many years, I expect to live for many more. Today, and for the rest of my life, I ask you to accept and honor me as Crone. And I wish to commit to you, my community and family, my intention as Crone to . . . " (Speak your intent.) The oldest woman present gives you a ball of yarn; she holds the end. You move around the circle, unwinding a long continuous thread into everyone's outstretched hands.

When you're done, ask everyone to stretch the yarn taut between their hands, close their eyes and think of something they would like to end." After a minute of silence, begin to move to your right around the circle, cutting the yarn between their hands and saying, in your own words: "I am She-Who-Holds-Her-Wise-Blood-Inside. I have crowned myself Crone and accepted the responsibility of giving death. I cut the thread. I set it free."

When you finish, invite each person to keep the yarn or to place it in a special basket, to be left outdoors as a give away.

To close, hum as before, asking the entire circle to join you. Thank the energies and attributes of the seven directions (inside, below, above, north, west, south, and east). Then, let there be feasting and dancing, music and pleasure, flowers and feathers, spring water and herbal wine, lit candles and lovely clothes. You have completed your menopausal years. You are truly Crone, a woman of wholeness.

* * * * *

Note: This ceremony marks the birth, the beginning, of your new identity as Crone. Most older women I spoke with felt they didn't fully settle into their new self image until the age of 60, or after their second Saturn return.

# Herbal References

"Common Herbs for Natural Health," Juliette Levy, Schocken, 1974
"Dictionary of Modern Herbalism," S. Mills, Healing Arts, 1988
"The Family Herbal," Barbara & P. Theiss, Healing Arts, 1989
"Guide to Medicinal Plants," P. Schauenberg & F. Paris, Keats, 1977
"Healing Wise," S. Weed, Ash Tree, 1989
"The Herb Book," John Lust, Bantam, 1974
"Herbs," R. Phillips & Nicky Fox, Random House, 1990
"Hygeia: A Woman's Herbal," Jeannine Parvati, Freestone, 1978
"Kings American Dispensatory," Eclectic Med. Pub., 1983
"Natural Healing in Gynecology," Rina Nissim, Pandora, 1984
"Nutritional Herbology," M. Pedersen, Pedersen Pub, 1987 • Avoid
    volume 2.
"The New Age Herbalist," R. Mabey with Gail Duff, M. McIntyre, Pamela
    Michael, J. Stevens, Gaia/Collier, 1988
"Phytotherapy Review," DJ Brown, in *Townsend Letter for Doctors*,
    May 1992
"Vitex: The Female Herb," C. Hobbs, Botanical, 1990

# Herbal Resources

Amrita Herbals • "From the fairies to you."
Rt. 1, Box 737, Floyd, VA 24380

Avena Botanicals • "Lovingly grown and wildcrafted."
PO Box 365, West Rockport, ME 04865

Blessed Herbs • "Serving the highest spirit in all."
Rt. 5, Box 1042, Ava, MO 65608 (dried, bulk botanicals)

Ryan Drum • "Exquisitely vital, vibrant dried herbs."
Waldron Island, WA 98297 (incredible kelp)

Green Terrestrial • "In co-creation with the devas."
Box 41, Rt 9W, Milton NY 12547

Herb Pharm • "Highest quality products available."
Box 116, Williams, OR 97544

Wish Garden Herbs • "Attention to detail."
PO Box 1304, Boulder, CO 80306

# Appendix 1
# Vitamins and Minerals
# For the Menopausal Years

Lists are arranged thusly: Most important sources, in decreasing order; then, other excellent sources.

**Vitamin A:** Vitamin A is formed in the liver from ingested carotenes. (See carotenes.) No plants contain vitamin A, but fish livers, animal livers, and liver oils do.

*Depleted by:* Coffee, alcohol, cortisone, mineral oil, fluorescent lights, liver "cleansing," excessive intake of iron, lack of protein.

**Vitamin B complex:** For healthy digestion, good liver function, emotional flexibility, less anxiety, sound sleep, milder hot flashes with less sweating, steady heart beat.

*Depleted by:* Coffee, alcohol, tobacco, sugar, raw oysters, ERT, birth control pills (deplete $B_6$ especially).

Sources of B vitamins: Whole grains, greens, organ meats (liver, kidneys, heart), sweet potatoes, carrots, molasses, nuts, bananas, avocados, grapes, pears; egg yolk, sardines, herring, salmon, crab, oysters, whey.

**Herbal Sources of B vitamins:** Red clover, parsley, oatstraw. See also specific B vitamins as follows.

**Vitamin $B_1$, Thiamine:** For emotional ease, strong nerves.

Sources of $B_1$, Thiamine: Asparagus, cauliflower, cabbage, kale, barley grass, spirulina, seaweeds, citrus fruit.

**Herbal Sources of $B_2$, Thiamine:** Peppermint, burdock, sage, yellow dock; alfalfa, red clover, fenugreek, raspberry leaves, nettles, catnip, watercress, yarrow, briar rose buds and rose hips.

**Vitamin $B_2$, Riboflavin:** For more energy, healthy skin, cancer prevention.

*Depleted by:* Hot flashes, crying jags, antibiotics, tranquilizers.

Sources of $B_2$, Riboflavin: Beans, greens, onions, seaweeds, spirulina, dairy products, mushrooms.

**Herbal Sources of $B_2$, Riboflavin:** Peppermint, alfalfa, parsley, echinacea, yellow dock, hops; dandelion, ginseng, dulse, kelp, fenugreek, rose hips, nettles.

**Vitamin $B_6$, Pyridoxine:** For improved immune functioning; especially needed if you are taking ERT.

Sources of Vitamin $B_6$, Pyridoxine: Baked potato with skin, broccoli, prunes, bananas, dried beans and lentils; all meats, poultry, fish.

**Vitamin B factor, Folic Acid:** For strong, flexible bones, easy nerves.
Sources of Folic Acid: Leafy greens.

**Herbal Sources of Folic Acid:** Nettles, alfalfa, parsley, sage, catnip,
peppermint, plantain, comfrey leaves, chickweed.

**Vitamin B factor, Niacin:** For relief of anxiety and depression,
decrease in headaches, reduction of blood cholesterol levels.

Sources of Niacin: Asparagus, spirulina, cabbage, bee pollen.

**Herbal Sources of Niacin:** Hops, raspberry leaf, red clover; slippery
elm, echinacea, licorice, rose hips, nettles, alfalfa, parsley.

**Bioflavonoids:** For healthy heart and blood vessels, fewer hot flashes
and night sweats, less menstrual bleeding, unlumpy breasts, less water
retention, less anxiety, less irritable nerves.

Sources of Bioflavonoids: Citrus pulp and rind.

**Herbal Sources of Bioflavonoids:** Buckwheat greens, blue green algae,
elder berries, hawthorn fruits, rose hips, horsetail, shepherd's purse,
chervil.

**Carotenes:** For a well-lubricated vagina, strong bones, protection
against cancer, healthy lungs and skin, strong vision, good digestion.

Sources of Carotenes: Carrots, cabbage, winter squash, sweet potatoes, dark leafy greens, apricots, spirulina, seaweeds.

**Herbal Sources of Carotenes:** Peppermint, yellow dock, uva ursi,
parsley, alfalfa, raspberry leaves, nettles, dandelion greens; kelp, green
onions, violet leaves, cayenne, paprika, lamb's quarters, sage, peppermint, chickweed, horsetail, black cohosh, rose hips.

**Vitamin C complex:** For less intense hot flashes, less insomnia and
night sweats, stronger bones, fewer headaches, better resistance to
infection, smoother emotions, less heart disease, rapid wound healing.
Your adrenals especially need the vitamin C complex during menopause.

*Depleted by:* Antibiotics, aspirin and other pain relievers, coffee,
stress, aging, smoking, baking soda, high fever.

Sources of Vitamin C: Fresh fruits and vegetables.

**Herbal Sources of Vitamin C:** Rose hips, yellow dock root, raspberry
leaf, red clover, hops; nettles, pine needles, dandelion greens, alfalfa,
echinacea, skullcap, plantain, parsley, cayenne, paprika.

**Vitamin D:** For very strong, very flexible bones, hormonal ease,
cancer prevention, regulation of glucose metabolism, reduction of risk
of adult onset diabetes.

*Depleted by:* Mineral oil used on the skin, frequent baths, sunscreens
with SPF 8 or higher.

Sources of Vitamin D: Sunlight, butter, egg yolk, cod liver oil; liver,

shrimp, fatty fish such as mackerel, sardines, herring, salmon, tuna.
**Herbal Sources of Vitamin D**: None; vitamin D is not found in plants.

**Vitamin E:** For milder hot flashes, fewer night sweats, protection
from cancer, fewer signs of aging, less wrinkles, moist vagina, strong
heart, freedom from arthritis.

*Depleted by*: Mineral oil, sulphates, ERT.

Sources of Vitamin E: Freshly ground whole grain flours, cold-pressed
vegetable oils; fresh nuts, leafy greens, kale, cabbage, asparagus.

**Herbal Sources of Vitamin E**: Alfalfa, rose hips, nettles, Dang Gui,
watercress, dandelion, seaweeds, wild seeds.

**Essential fatty acids** (EFAs), including GLA, omega-6, and omega-3:
For healthy heart, less severe hot flashes, strong nerves, strong bones,
fully functioning endocrine glands, fewer wrinkles.

Sources of EFAs: Safflower oil, wheat germ oil.

**Herbal Sources of EFAs**: All wild plants (but very few cultivated plants)
contain EFAs; purslane is notably high. Commercial sources include
seed oils of flax, evening primrose, black currant, and borage.

**Folic Acid:** See vitamin B factor, folic acid.

**Vitamin K:** For less menstrual flooding.

*Depleted by*: X-rays, radiation, air pollution, enemas, frozen foods,
antibiotics, rancid fats, aspirin.

Sources of Vitamin K: Healthy intestinal bacteria produce vitamin
K; green leafy vegetables, yogurt, egg yolk, blackstrap molasses.

**Herbal Sources of Vitamin K**: Nettles, alfalfa, kelp, green tea.

**Boron:** For strong, flexible bones.

Sources of Boron: Organic fruits, vegetables, nuts.

**Herbal Sources of Boron**: All organic garden weeds including chickweed, purslane, nettles, dandelion, yellow dock.

**Calcium:** For sound sleep, dense bones, calm heart, strong muscles,
less irritable nerves, lower blood pressure, sound blood vessels, regular
heart beat, freedom from depression and headaches, less bloating,
fewer mood fluctuations.

*Depleted by*: Coffee, sugar, salt, alcohol, cortisone, enemas, too
much phosphorus.

Sources of Calcium: Dark green leaves, yogurt; nuts and seeds (especially tahini), seaweed, vegetables (such as sweet potatoes or cabbage),
dried beans, whole grains, whey, salmon, tuna, sardines, shellfish.

**Herbal Sources of Calcium**: Valerian, kelp, nettles, horsetail, peppermint; sage, uva ursi, yellow dock, chickweed, red clover, oatstraw,
parsley, black currant leaf, raspberry leaf, plantain leaf/seed, borage,
dandelion leaf, amaranth leaves, lamb's quarter.

**Chromium:** For less fatigue and lots of energy, fewer mood swings, more stable blood sugar levels, higher HDL. Reduces risk of adult onset diabetes.

*Depleted by*: White sugar.

Sources of Chromium: Barley grass, bee pollen, prunes, nuts, mushrooms, liver, beets, whole wheat.

**Herbal Sources of Chromium:** Oatstraw, nettles, red clover, catnip, dulse, wild yam, yarrow, horsetail; black cohosh, licorice, echinacea, valerian, sarsaparilla.

**Copper:** For supple skin, healthy hair, strong muscles, easy nerves, less water retention, less menstrual flooding, lower blood cholesterol.

Sources of Copper: Seafood, organically grown grains, beans, nuts, leafy greens, seaweeds, bittersweet chocolate.

**Herbal Sources of Copper:** Skullcap, sage, horsetail; chickweed.

**Iodine:** For fewer breast lumps, less fatigue, strong thyroid and liver.

Sources of Iodine: Seafood, seaweed, sea salt, spinach, beets, mushrooms.

**Herbal sources of Iodine:** Kelp, parsley, celery, sarsaparilla.

**Iron:** For fewer hot flashes, less menstrual flooding, fewer headaches, better sleep with fewer night sweats, easier nerves, more energy, less dizziness.

*Depleted by*: Coffee, black tea, enemas, alcohol, aspirin, carbonated drinks, lack of protein, too much dairy.

Sources of Iron: Leafy greens, molasses, dried fruit (cherries, raisins), liver, yellow/orange/red vegetables, bittersweet chocolate; whole wheat, oatmeal, brown rice, mushrooms, potatoes, honey, seaweeds, canned salmon, sardines.

**Herbal Sources of Iron:** Chickweed, kelp, burdock, catnip, horsetail, *Althea* root, milk thistle seed, uva ursi, dandelion leaf/root; yellow dock root, Dang Gui, black cohosh, echinacea, plantain leaves, nettles, licorice, valerian, fenugreek, sarsaparilla, peppermint.

**Magnesium:** For deeper sleep, less anxiety, easier nerves, flexible bones and arteries, lower cholesterol, lower blood pressure, stronger heart, more energy, less fatigue, fewer headaches/migraines.

*Depleted by*: Hot flashes, night sweats, crying jags, alcohol, chemical diuretics, enemas, antibiotics, "soft" water, excessive fat intake.

Sources of Magnesium: Leafy greens, seaweeds, nuts, whole grains, yogurt, cheese; potatoes, corn, peas, squash.

**Herbal Sources of Magnesium:** Oatstraw, licorice, kelp, nettles, dulse, burdock, chickweed, *Althea* root, horsetail; sage, raspberry leaf, red clover, valerian, yellow dock, dandelion greens, carrot tops, parsley, evening primrose.

**Manganese:** For keen hearing, flexible bones, reduction of dizziness, prevention of diabetes.

*Depleted by:* Chemical fertilizers used agriculturally.

Sources of Manganese: Any leaf or seed from a plant grown in healthy soil; seaweeds.

**Herbal Sources of Manganese:** Raspberry leaf, uva ursi, chickweed, milk thistle, yellow dock; ginseng, wild yam, hops, catnip, echinacea, horsetail, kelp, nettles, dandelion.

**Molybdenum:** For fewer hot flashes, prevention of anemia.

Sources of Molybdenum: Organically raised dairy products, legumes, grains, leafy greens.

**Herbal Sources of Molybdenum:** Nettles, dandelion greens, sage, oatstraw, fenugreek, raspberry leaves, red clover, horsetail, chickweed, seaweeds.

**Nickel:** For milder hot flashes, easy nerves.

Sources of Nickel: Chocolate, nuts, dried beans, cereals.

**Herbal Sources of Nickel:** Alfalfa, red clover, oatstraw, fenugreek.

**Phosphorus:** For strong, flexible bones, more energy.

*Depleted by:* Antacids.

Sources of Phosphorus: Whole grains, seeds, nuts.

**Herbal Sources of Phosphorus:** Peppermint, yellow dock, milk thistle, fennel, hops, chickweed; nettles, dandelion, parsley, dulse, red clover.

**Potassium:** For more energy, less fatigue, less water retention, firm stools, easy weight loss, steady heart beat, lower blood pressure, better digestion.

*Depleted by:* Frequent hot flashes with sweating, night sweats, coffee, sugar, salt, alcohol, enemas, vomiting, diarrhea, chemical diuretics, dieting.

Sources of Potassium: Celery, cabbage, peas, parsley, broccoli, peppers, carrots, potato skins, eggplant, whole grains, pears, citrus, seaweeds.

**Herbal Sources of Potassium:** Sage, catnip, hops, dulse, peppermint, skullcap, kelp, red clover; horsetail, nettles, borage, plantain.

**Selenium:** For clear vision, slower aging, strong immune response, less irritability, more energy, healthy hair/nails/teeth, less cardiovascular disease.

Sources of Selenium: Dairy products, seaweeds, grains, garlic, liver, kidneys, fish, shellfish.

**Herbal Sources of Selenium:** Catnip, milk thistle, valerian, dulse, black cohosh, ginseng; uva ursi, hops, echinacea, kelp, raspberry leaf, rose buds and hips, hawthorn berries, fenugreek, sarsaparilla, yellow dock.

**Silicon:** For strong, flexible bones, less irritable nerves.

Sources of Silicon: Unrefined grains, root vegetables, spinach, leeks.

**Herbal Sources of Silicon/Silica:** Horsetail, dulse, echinacea, cornsilk, burdock, oatstraw, licorice, chickweed; uva ursi, sarsaparilla.

**Sulfur:** For relaxed muscles, soft skin, healthy nerves, strong liver, glossy hair.

Sources of Sulfur: Eggs, dairy products, cabbage family plants, onions, garlic, parsley, watercress.

**Herbal Sources of Sulfur:** Sage, nettles, plantain, horsetail.

**Zinc:** For slower aging, better digestion, stronger bones, healthy skin, cancer prevention, increased sex drive.

*Depleted by:* Alcohol, air pollution, ERT.

Sources of Zinc: Pumpkin seeds, oysters, spirulina.

**Herbal Sources of Zinc:** Skullcap, sage, wild yam, chickweed, echinacea, nettles, dulse, milk thistle; sarsaparilla.

# Appendix 2

# Strong Bone Stew
*Serves 3-4*

In a large, heavy-bottomed pot, heat 2 tablespoons/30 ml **olive oil**. Sauté in the warm oil 1 cup/250 ml organically grown **chopped onions**, 1-3 cloves **chopped garlic**, and 1 cup/250 ml **quartered mushrooms**. When onions are soft, add 1 quart/liter **vegetable stock** (or water), and bring to a boil.

Then add 1 cup/250 ml each of at least four of these organically grown vegetables, cubed, unpeeled: **sweet potato, carrot, turnip, winter squash, potato, parsnip, burdock/gobo**. Also add ½ cup/125 ml **dried wakame seaweed**, cut small. Simmer for 45 minutes, adding more water or broth if needed.

While the stew simmers, mix together in a large measuring cup or bowl: 2 tablespoons/30 ml **miso**, 2 teaspoons/10 ml **tamari**, ⅓ cup/80 ml **tahini**, 2 tablespoons/30 ml **peanut or almond butter**, 1 tablespoon/15 ml **cronewort vinegar**. (See page 192.)

Just before serving, ladle enough hot broth into the measuring cup or bowl to make a mixture thin enough to pour into the stew. Add this mix and 1 cake **tofu**, cubed, to your stewpot. Continue to cook on very low heat for 5 minutes. Serve hot, with whole grain bread or brown rice.

*Thirteen great calcium-rich foods all in one pot. My thanks to "New Recipes from Moosewood" for sparking the creation of this delight.*

# Fruit Fix

Simmer together in 8-10 cups/2000-2500 ml **water**:
1 pound/450 grams pitted **dates**
1 pound/450 grams dried **figs**
1 pound/450 grams pitted **prunes**
1½ pounds/675 grams **raisins**
When soft, mash together (or put in food processor) and add
2-4 tablespoons **rose hip powder**. Use this calcium-rich, estrogen-enhancing spread in place of jams and jellies. Try it on a whole wheat cracker when you think you want a cookie.

*To relieve constipation, cook in prune juice instead of water.*

# How To Make an Herbal Infusion

A *tea* is a small amount of fresh or dried herb brewed for a short time. An **infusion** is a large amount of dried (not fresh) herb brewed for a long time. An infusion extracts more nutrients than a tincture and more medicinal qualities (and nutrients) than a tea. Most infusions are short-lived; they stay good for only two or three days.

Prepare infusions in pint/half-liter and quart/liter jars with tight lids. A teapot is not as good, but acceptable.

Usual dose of infusion is 1-2 cups/250-500 ml a day, taken hot, chilled, or at room temperature. Infusions may be seasoned with sweeteners, tamari, milk, or any other additions that please your taste. Infusions can be used as soup stocks, bath waters, hair rinses, facial washes, and so on.

## Summary of Infusion Data

| Plant Part | Amount | Jar/Water | Length of Infusion |
|---|---|---|---|
| **Roots/barks** | 1 oz/30 g. | **pint/500 ml** | 8 hours minimum |
| **Leaves** | 1 oz/30 g. | **quart/liter** | 4 hours minimum |
| **Flowers** | 1 oz/30 g. | **quart/liter** | 2 hours maximum |
| **Seeds/berries** | 1 oz/30 g. | **pint/500 ml** | 30 minutes maximum |

## Bonny Bony Brew

**Nettle** (*Urtica dioica*), 1 ounce/30 grams, dry
**Horsetail** (*Equisetum arvense*), 1 tablespoon/2 grams, dry
**Sage** (*Salvia officinalis*), 1 tablespoon/2 grams, dry

Crush sage between palms and drop into a quart/liter container with the other two herbs. Fill jar with water just off the boil, cap tightly, and sit in a cozy corner to brew for at least four hours (overnight is fine). Strain; drink as is or heat and add honey. Also nice iced. You can substitute red clover or oatstraw or raspberry for the nettles.

*Each cup contributes as much calcium as a cup of milk.*

# How To Make an Herbal Tincture

Fresh plant material steeped in alcohol makes alkaloid-rich (but nutrient-poor) herbal remedies called *tinctures*. If you cannot find the fresh herb, you may use dried herbs, but in my experience, only dried roots, seeds, and berries are worth the effort. (Flowers and leaves lose too much in the drying.) Tinctures remain effective for long periods of time and are easily transported. Vinegar does not extract the same properties from plants as alcohol.

To tincture: Identify and pick the plant. Chop the plant material coarsely; do not wash. Fill any size jar with the plant material, then pour 100 proof vodka (or grain alcohol) over it, filling the jar to the top. Cap tightly. Label with date and name of plant. Your tincture will be ready to use in six weeks but can sit there for as long as you wish.

## Summary of Tincture Proportions

• Tincture **one ounce/30 grams fresh** plant material in approximately **one ounce/30 ml** spirit for 6 weeks.

• Tincture **one ounce/30 grams dried** plant material in **five ounces/ 150 ml** spirit for 6 weeks.

## Jiffy Motherwort Tonics

Put fresh flowering motherwort (*Leonurus cardiaca*) through a juicer. Mix 4 tablespoons/60 ml of this fresh motherwort juice with:

**vodka**, 4 tablespoons/60 ml *or*
**honey**, 1 cup/250 ml *or*
**vinegar**, ½ cup/125 ml.

Motherwort tincture takes six weeks. If you're in a hurry, try this. But put up some tincture, too. This doesn't work as well.

*Keep refrigerated.*

# How to Make an Herbal Vinegar

Natural vinegars, such as apple cider vinegar, wine vinegar, rice vinegar, and so on, are especially effective mediums for extracting the mineral richness of plants. Some alkaloidal components may dissolve in vinegar as well. Fill a jar with fresh leaves, roots, flowers. Then fill with vinegar, label, and cap. Use fresh plant material only. Do beware vinegar's ability to corrode metal; use plastic lids or corks for your herbal vinegars (or put a piece of plastic wrap over the jar before screwing on a metal lid). Ready to use in six weeks.

# Old Sour Puss Mineral Mix

☞ **Yellow Dock** (*Rumex*) leaves/roots
☞ **Dandelion** (*Taraxacum*) leaves/roots
☞ **Plantain** (*Plantago*) leaves
☞ **Nettle** (*Urtica*) leaves
☞ **Raspberry** (*Rubus*) leaves/canes/berries
☞ **Cronewort/Mugwort** (*Artemisia vulgaris*) leaves
☞ **Comfrey** (*Symphytum*) leaves/flower stalks
☞ **Red Clover** (*Trifolium pratense*) blossoms
☞ Clean **eggshells**, or clean bones may also be used

Completely fill a quart/liter jar with one (or more) of these calcium-rich herbs. Use only fresh plant material.

Pour apple cider vinegar over the herbs until the jar is full. Cover with a plastic lid and let sit for six weeks.

Use this calcium-rich vinegar as a refreshing drink before meals by mixing a tablespoon/30 ml in up to a cup of water. For the hardy, and those in need of iron, add a tablespoon/30 ml of molasses. (Adds 150 mg more calcium, too.)

Also great added to soups and bean dishes, and as a salad dressing.

*Vinegar has the amazing ability to dissolve calcium (and other minerals) and hold it in solution, ready for your ingestion and assimilation. A tablespoon/30 ml of this vinegar will supply about 150-200 mg calcium. Taken before or with your meals, this vinegar increases the digestibilty of the minerals in your entire meal.*

# Menopausal Root Brew

**Black Cohosh** (*Cimicifuga racemosa*) roots
**Black Haw** or Cramp Bark (*Viburnum prunifolium, V. opulis*)
**Burdock** (*Arctium lappa*) roots
**Dandelion** (*Taraxacum off.*) roots
**Devil's Club** (*Oplopanax horridum*) root bark
**False Unicorn** (*Chamaelirium luteum*) roots
**Ginseng** (*Panax*) roots
**Osha** (*Ligusticum porterii*) roots
**Peony** (*Paeonia*) roots
**Rehmannia** (*R. glutinosa*) roots
**Sarsaparilla** (*Smilax* species) roots
**Spikenard** (*Aralia* species) roots
**Wild Ginger** (*Asarum canadensis*) roots
**Wild Yam** (*Dioscorea* species) roots
**Yellow Dock** (*Rumex crispus*) roots

Gather fresh any *three* of these hormone-rich roots (root bark). Substitute local species as desired. (There are many varieties of yellow dock, wild yam, and wild ginger to choose from, for example.)

Nearly fill any jar with chopped pieces of these fresh roots. You may add one dried **Ginseng** or **Dang Gui** root, if desired. Fill jar to the top with 100 proof vodka. Let sit for six weeks. Then use 10-30 drops, once or twice a day, in a cup of water or garden sage tea. This brew will help you through your menopausal climax years and into a healthy, happy Cronehood.

# How To Make an Herbal Glycerine Macerate

Glycerine, a by-product of soap-making, is used to extract hormonal precursors and glycosides from plants. You can buy glycerine at the drugstore. The procedure for macerating plants in glycerin is exactly the same as the procedure for making a tincture. Use fresh plants only. Fill a jar with your plant material; completely cover with glycerine diluted 1:1, 1:2, or 1:3 with water; and macerate, tightly capped, for at least six weeks.

# Dong Quai/Dang Gui Tonic

**Dang Gui** (*Angelica sinensis*), 1 ounce/30 grams dried root
**Burdock** (*Arctium lappa*), ¼ ounce/7 grams dried root
**Peony** (*Paeonia off.*), ¼ ounce/7 grams dried root
**Dandelion** (*Taraxucum off.*), ¼ ounce/7 grams dried root

Put your roots in a pint/60 ml jar and fill it to the top with 100 proof vodka or apple cider vinegar. Cap well and label. Wait at least six weeks before using. If you have fresh burdock, dandelion, or peony root (yes, it's the one in your garden), substitute 1 ounce/30 grams fresh for ¼ ounce/7 grams dried. To take, put a dropperful into a cup of water or fenugreek seed (*Trigonella foenum-graecum*) tea. CAUTION: Grannies say there's a baby in every cup of fenugreek.

# Menopausal First Aid

*Eases hot flashes, palpitations, insomnia, night sweats, and anxiety.*

**Chickweed** (*Stellaria media*) leaf and flower tincture
**Motherwort** (*Leonurus cardiaca*) tincture of flowering tops

Combine equal parts of these tinctures in a one-ounce/30 ml dropper bottle. Use 10-20 drops, as needed, in some water or, better yet, a cup of sage infusion or fenugreek tea.

# Easy Homemade Yogurt

1 gallon/4 liters **milk**, any kind
1 cup/250 ml **plain yogurt** with *active cultures*

Heat milk over a small flame in a non-metal pot. Stir and feel frequently. When milk feels just a little warm (105°F/37°C), remove from heat. Put yogurt into a glass bowl or quart/liter measuring cup. Add a cup/250 ml of warmed milk. Stir well. Pour this mix into a one-gallon glass jar. (Ask a local restaurant or deli for one.) Add all the rest of the warmed milk, stir well with a wooden spoon, cap, and set to rest in a warm place (100-110°F/37-39°C) for 8-24 hours. The longer it sits, the easier it will be to digest. Keeps refrigerated for four to six weeks.

# Springing Soup
### serves 4

To 8 cups/2 liters **water** or vegetable broth, add fresh **nettle greens**, 2 cups/500 ml, and fresh **horsetail**, one handful. Chop 4 **potatoes** and add. Bring to a boil and simmer until potatoes are done. Garnish with wild onions finely minced.

# Oat Bath

Make 2 quarts/liters of oatstraw infusion. Add to a hot bath and soak your tensions away. Or put a handful of rolled oats in a kitchen towel, tie it closed loosely, and toss it in a hot bath. When it softens, rub it down all your limbs, from thigh to toes and shoulder to fingertips.

# Peel Power

*A spoonful of bioflavonoid-rich citrus peels is delicious this way.*

Juice **2 organic oranges** and 1 **organic lemon.** Cut the peels (together with inner membranes) into very thin slivers of any length. Heat with 1 cup/250 ml of **honey** until it just boils. Pour immediately into jar, filling it to the brim. Cap. You can use this the very next day, but it does improve with age.

# Plantain Ointment

Collect fresh, dark green plantain leaves. Immediately chop them coarsely and put into a clean, dry jar. Don't quite fill the jar. Pour enough **olive oil** over the leaves to come to the top of the jar. Cap well. Label. Leave on a wooden counter for six weeks. (Some of the oil may leak out.) Squeeze oil from leaves. Add 1 tablespoon/1 gram beeswax per ounce/30 ml oil and heat gently. Pour in jar; cool.

# How To Make an Herbal Compress or Poultice

Any fresh herb chewed or crushed and applied to the body is a **poultice**. A **compress** uses dried herbs. To make a compress, first make an herbal infusion. Then strain the liquid off the plant material and put the wet plants in a cloth. Apply, hot or cold, to the painful area. Dip the cloth in the liquid as needed to keep the compress moist.

# Glossary

**Adaptogenic**: An agent that helps us adapt, especially to stress. Adaptogens tend to be tonifying and nourishing, rather than stimulating.

**Adenomatous hyperplasia**: See hyperplasia.

**Bioflavonoids**: Brightly colored substances frequently found in fruits and vegetables in association with ascorbic acid (vitamin C). Also known as vitamin P. Bioflavonoids are required for absorption of vitamin C. Citrin, hesperidin, rutin, flavones, and flavonals are bioflavonoids.

**Chakra**: Sanskrit word meaning "wheel." The chakras of the human body are energy wheels or energy centers.

**Corpus luteum**: A mound of yellow, hormone-producing tissue that occurs in the wall of the ovary when (and where) an egg has just been released. It encourages production of progesterone.

**Endometrial hyperplasia**: Overgrowth of the lining of the uterus. See hyperplasia.

**Endometriosis**: Endometrial tissue growing somewhere other than inside the uterus, where it belongs. It may cause menstrual pain, midcycle spotting, flooding, and infertility, but it is unlikely to be life-threatening or cancerous. Endometriosis is progesterone-dependent, and usually disappears after menopause.

**Endometrium**: The lining of the uterus. It grows each cycle and is shed in menstruation.

**ERT**: Estrogen replacement therapy. A treatment urged on menopausal women based on the assumption that menopause is an "estrogen deficiency disease" and that mid-life women need to have their "lost" estrogen replaced. ERT causes uterine cancer so frequently that women are advised to have an endometrial biopsy (a painful, invasive process) annually while taking ERT. The connection between ERT and breast cancer is also established and yearly mammograms are advised for those taking ERT.

**Estrogen**: A group of more than two dozen closely related steroidal hormones produced primarily by the ovaries, adrenals, fat cells, testicles, placenta and fetus. *Estropipate, estrone, estradiol,* and *estriol* are forms of estrogen. Estrogen levels in most 60-year-old women are indistinguishable from estrogen levels in most 40-year-old women. Menopause is not a result of estrogen deficiency. High levels of estrogen are thought to be responsible for many reproductive cancers. *Estrogenic*, adj.

**Fibroid:** A benign growth in the uterus or breast.

**Flavonoids:** See Bioflavonoids.

**FSH:** Follicle stimulating hormone. Produced primarily by the pituitary, FSH triggers ovulation. Levels of FSH rise dramatically in the menopausal years and remain high post-menopausally.

**GLA:** Gamma linoleic acid; an essential fatty acid, that is, a fat that *must* be consumed to maintain good health. Flaxseed oil contains linoleic and linolenic acids; most vegetable oils contain only linolenic.

**Glycoside:** A carbohydrate that breaks down into a sugar and a non-sugar. Plant glycosides affect hormone-producing tissues powerfully.

**HRT:** Hormone replacement therapy; that is, the replacement of both progesterone and estrogen by way of pills or injections.

**Hyperplasia:** Literally an increase in the number of cells in an area or organ. Menopausal women who take supplemental estrogen (ERT) frequently experience **adenomatous hyperplasia** and **endometrial hyperplasia**. Hyperplasia itself is not cancer and does not create cancer, but ERT *is* undeniably linked to uterine cancer.

**Hysterectomy:** Removal (-ectomy) of the uterus (hyster).

**LH:** Luteinizing hormone; produced primarily by the pituitary. In combination with FSH, LH stimulates the ovaries to secrete estrogen, which in turn triggers ovulation. LH is also responsible for changing the ovum follicle into the corpus luteum. LH levels rise dramatically during the menopausal years, and stay elevated through post-menopause. Overproduction of melatonin by the pineal gland can stop release of LH.

**Luteal phase:** The thirteen-day interval between ovulation and menstruation. There is no luteal phase if pregnancy occurs.

**Moxibustion:** Burning (com*bustion*) of *moxa* (dried "wool" of *Artemisia vulgaris*). Moxibustion warms, eases pain, and tonifies the energy.

**Palpitations:** A pounding, racing heart. See also tachycardia.

**Polyp:** A small growth emerging from a mucous membrane surface such as the cervix, vagina, or rectum.

**Precursor:** Comes before, or is easily transformed into. Glycosides and bioflavonoids are hormonal precursors.

**Progesterone:** A group of pro-gestational steroidal hormones primarily produced by the corpus luteum, adrenals, and placenta. Progesterone is produced when ovulation occurs. As ovulation slows and ceases during the menopausal years, progesterone levels fall. Most 60-year-old women have little or no progesterone. It is a critical hormone in bone formation.

**Progestin:** Synthetic progesterone given as part of HRT may be called *progestin, progestogen,* or *progestagen.* Natural progesterone is sometimes called progestin, too.

**Prostaglandins:** Hormone-like fatty acids that act in many ways: they influence hormone production, tonify smooth muscles (heart, uterus, intestines), and nourish the autonomic and central nervous systems.

**Phytosterols:** Hormones (sterols or steroids) found in plants (phyto).

**Saponins:** Soap-like substances found in plants. Saponins emulsify (combine oil and water) like soap, thus improving the body's absorption of hormones (fat-soluble substances). They also increase the permeability of cellular membranes, hastening and encouraging the absorption of all nutrients and the death of unwanted bacteria.

**Solar plexus:** The sun (solar) center (plexus). This chakra is associated with digestion, the liver and kidneys, feelings of self-worth and personal power, and bright yellow flowers like dandelion and sunflower.

**Tachycardia:** Literally "speedy heart"; very rapid heart beats, often accompanied by breathlessness, and a lightheaded sensation. Tachycardia occurs in healthy people during strenuous exercise. Tachycardia in a resting state may be due to overuse of coffee, fever, heart disease, or menopausal hot flashes.

**Yang:** Oriental term referring to warm, bright, expanded, active energy; originally, the sunny side of the river.

**Yin:** Oriental term referring to cool, dark, concentrated, meditative energy; originally, the shaded side of the river.

# Index